HARRI ANGELL

PILATES
FOR LIVING

HARRI ANGELL

PILATES
FOR LIVING

Get stronger, fitter and healthier for an active later life

BLOOMSBURY SPORT

LONDON • OXFORD • NEW YORK • NEW DELHI • SYDNEY

BLOOMSBURY SPORT
Bloomsbury Publishing Plc
50 Bedford Square, London, WC1B 3DP, UK

BLOOMSBURY, BLOOMSBURY SPORT and the Diana logo are trademarks of Bloomsbury Publishing Plc

First published in Great Britain 2018

A catalogue record for this book is available from the British Library

Library of Congress Cataloguing-in-Publication data has been applied for

ISBN: Paperback: 9781472947789 ePDF: 9781472947765

2 4 6 8 10 9 7 5 3 1

Designed by Susan McIntyre
Typeset in 11pt Myriad Pro Light Condensed
Printed and bound in China by Toppan Leefung Printing

Bloomsbury Publishing Plc makes every effort to ensure that the papers used in the manufacture of our books are natural, recyclable products made from wood grown in well-managed forests. Our manufacturing processes conform to the environmental regulations of the country of origin.

To find out more about our authors and books visit www.bloomsbury.com and sign up for our newsletters

Contents

Introduction 7

Chapter 1   Joseph Pilates: a brief history 11

Chapter 2   What Pilates can do for us as we age 15

Chapter 3   What is Pilates? The Pilates principles 21

Chapter 4   Equipment 25

Chapter 5   Postural alignment for living 29

Chapter 6   Breathing 39

Chapter 7   Gentle warm-up exercises for everyone 41

Chapter 8   Balance 55

Chapter 9   Foot health and strengthening exercises 59

Chapter 10 Mat Pilates exercises 67

Chapter 11 Post-activity stretches 181

Chapter 12 Three 20-minute routines – all levels 189

Chapter 13 The healing power of Pilates for body and mind 195

Chapter 14 Finding a mat Pilates class and what to look for 201

Glossary 203

About the author 204

Acknowledgements 204

Index 205

Terms in **bold and italics** are defined in the Glossary (page 203)

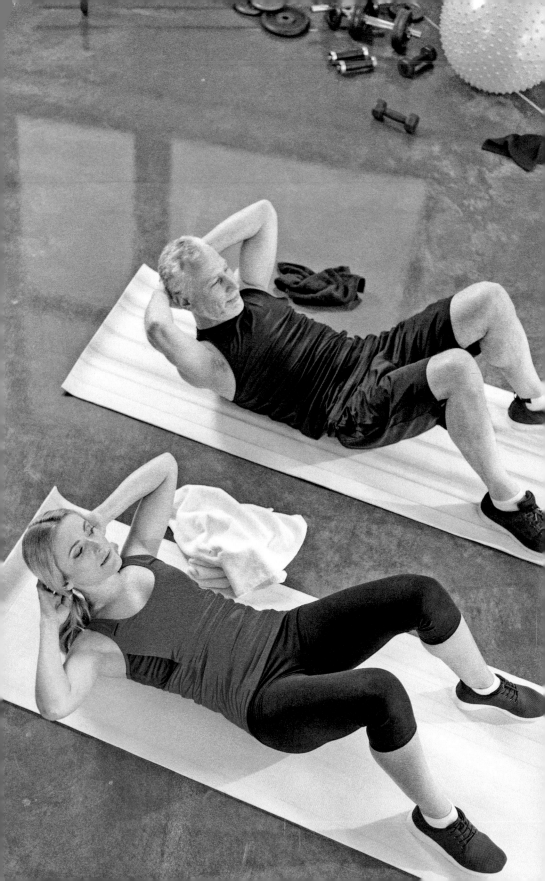

Introduction

Ageing is a natural, gradual process that happens to us all – there's nothing we can do to stop it. But we can slow it down. This book will show you how to do just that and build a foundation for successful future living.

Whatever your age, mat Pilates will improve your strength, coordination, mobility, flexibility, breathing, balance, concentration and general wellbeing. Your posture will improve as well. This will not only prevent aches and pains but also lift your spirits as you learn to stand up straighter, lengthen through the spine and embrace, head-on, those advancing years. To my mind, there is absolutely no point in dwelling on the negative aspect of the ageing process. We all know what happens to us both mentally and physically as we grow older, but we don't necessarily know how to challenge those inevitable changes.

Whether you've just hit your 40s or are heading for 70-plus, you can make those years ahead healthy, happy and fulfilling ones. Frailty, which can creep up on us in varying degrees from middle age onwards, is largely reversible. My guess is that you've picked up this book because you've decided that as the years progress you want to keep active and healthy, as I do.

There's so much emphasis in today's world on the negative aspects of growing older. Anti-ageing marketeers ply us with products and promises. As the decades fly by faster and faster, the inevitable starts to happen, you feel frail: 'I'm just getting old', you say, and settle for it. Well, I'm here to tell you to forget your age. Instead, concentrate more on living your life and keeping as fit and active as you can. There's no rule that says we have to stop walking long distances or playing golf or tennis once we reach a certain age. And by the same token, there's no rule that says you shouldn't start new activities once you've reached that certain age. I know many people who have taken up running in their 50s and 60s. There are no rules. Pilates is a marvellous, life-enhancing form of exercise, whatever your age, fitness level or ability. Trust me when I say it could just change your life for the better.

Are you considering a walking holiday but unsure whether you could manage those hills? Practise the exercises in this book and you will certainly be up for it. Do you dream of taking up new physical hobbies? Then go through the exercises in this book and you will be ready both mentally and physically to start taking on an exciting new challenge.

I know. I'm in my 50s and I run marathons, I cycle, walk long distances, teach Pilates, lift weights and I never intend to stop.

By practising Pilates a few times a week, I promise that you will feel the difference as your body gains strength and flexibility. You'll start to

> We retire too early and we die too young, our prime of life should be in the 70s and old age should not come until we are almost 100.
>
> Joseph Pilates, *Return to Life Through Contrology*

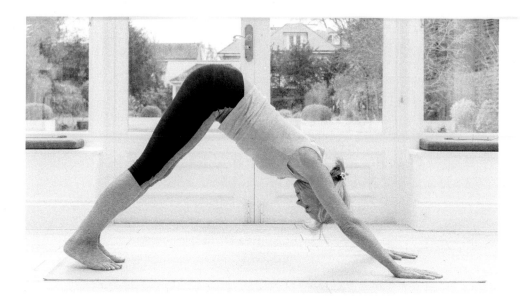

feel more confident as well. You might even notice that your body shape changes, you sleep better and you feel more mentally alert.

You'll find a range of exercises in this book to suit all sorts of fitness ability; so don't be intimidated if you haven't done anything like this before. We all have to start somewhere! There's a 'Starter Pack' chapter on page 68 if you're nervous or unsure of your ability – so called because it contains a little bit of everything, the basic things to get you going. In addition, there is a chapter on balance, which is a very important skill to continue to develop as we age or we can become more frail or prone to falling. You'll find a chapter on looking after feet and exercises to improve foot health – all this before you even get to the main Pilates exercises. So there is something for absolutely everyone.

If you have any musculoskeletal problems, medical conditions or aches and pains, these will be addressed – and Chapter 7 includes notes on knee and hip replacements, breast surgery and arthritis. If you do suffer from any serious problems or have recently undergone surgery, always seek advice from your medical practitioner before attempting any of the exercises.

While nearly all the exercises and some of the earlier chapters in this book stand alone, the postural alignment information in Chapter 5 will give you the components you need to get the most out of your regular practice. Even before you attempt the exercises, by applying some of the simple techniques outlined in Chapter 5, you can begin to improve your posture as you go about your everyday life, with the eventual effect of feeling years younger. You will begin to notice a difference quite quickly.

> Physical fitness is the first requisite of happiness. Our interpretation of physical fitness is the attainment and maintenance of a uniformly developed body with a sound mind fully capable of naturally, easily and satisfactorily performing our many and varied daily tasks with spontaneous zest and pleasure.
>
> Joseph Pilates, *Return to Life Through Contrology*

Each of the exercises and some of the chapters in this book start with a brief explanation of the specific benefits to us as we age. I always like to know why I'm doing an exercise to fully understand how it works – so where possible and at the risk of repetition there are explanatory notes. Not only will you learn how to perform the exercise but also why you need to do it and how it helps to improve your fitness levels. This will also enhance your body awareness. As we grow older, we tend to lose touch with our bodies. We can begin to feel weaker and so less able. It's important to reconnect with our bodies as this gives us a better sense of self and increases confidence, something that can diminish as the years advance.

My intention is to show you in the simplest, safest and most practical way how to practise these exercises in order to gain maximum benefit. If you feel discomfort, it goes without saying that you should stop – you will recognize the difference between working those muscles hard and something feeling not quite right. Listen to your body, work within your ability, understand the reasoning behind the exercises and follow the instructions, and you can't go wrong.

In addition, throughout the book you will find motivational case studies from both men and women at different stages of life who use Pilates, some of them my clients. There is also informative advice from professionals who advocate Pilates to alleviate specific conditions that can creep up on us as we age. Plus you'll find lots of inspirational quotes from the master himself, Joseph Pilates.

Good luck and let me know how you get on!

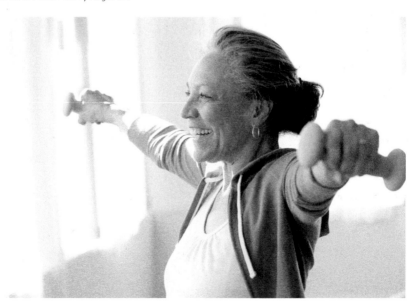

Chapter 1

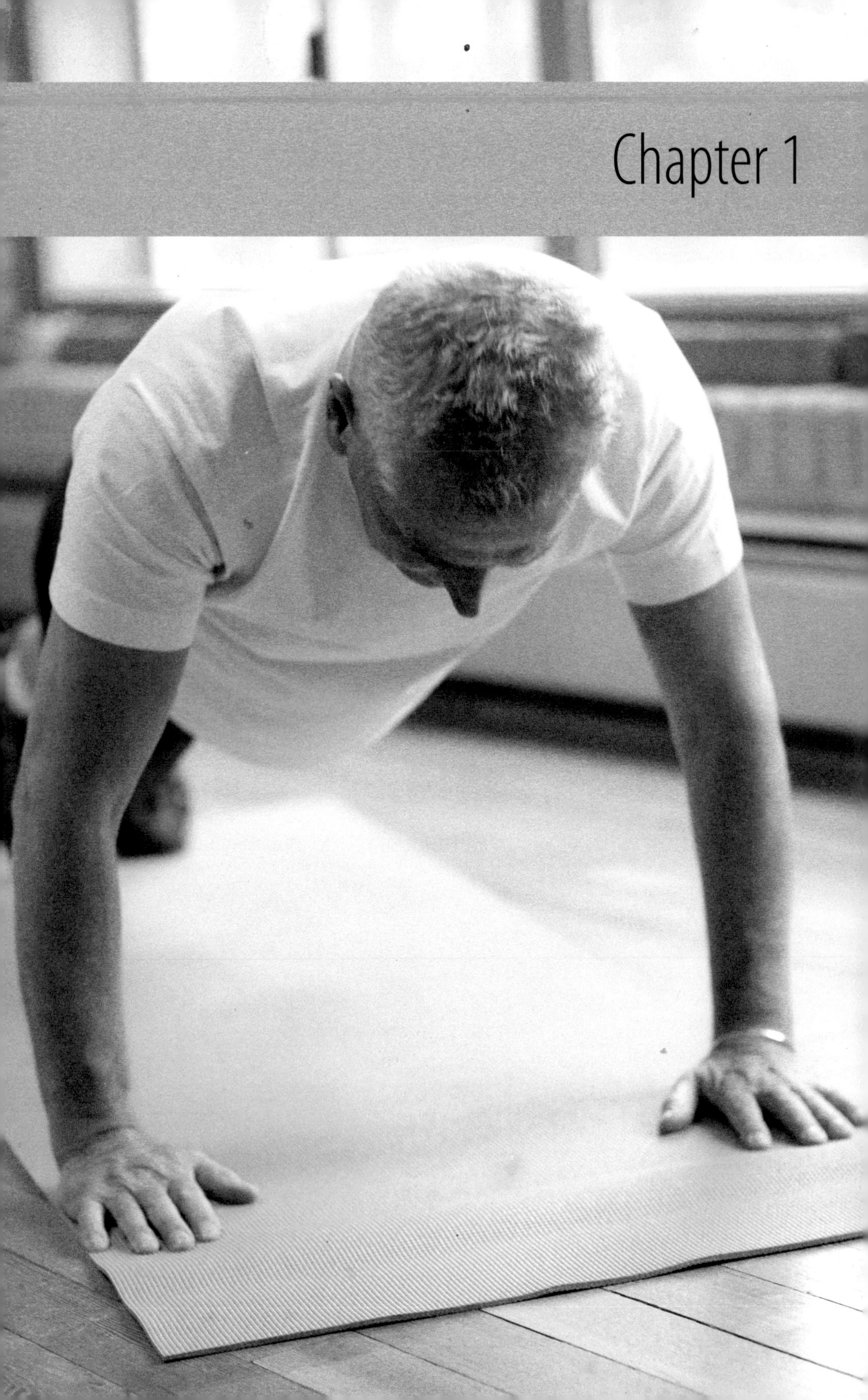

Joseph Pilates: a brief history

Joseph Hubertus Pilates was born in 1883 in Mönchengladbach, Germany, and the second of nine children. As a child, raised in poverty, he suffered from rickets, asthma and rheumatic fever. Growing up he became frustrated by his frailty so started to explore ways to increase his physical fitness and improve his health. Leaving his sickly childhood behind, he became a gymnast, skier, boxer, diver and bodybuilder, while also studying self-defence and meditation. As his body developed tone and shape, he even modelled for anatomy charts, so well defined were his muscles.

In 1912 Joseph Pilates moved to England and was employed to teach self-defence to members of the British Police Force and Army; some biographies also claim that he was a circus performer at the same time.

When World War I broke out he was interned in Knockaloe Camp for German civilians on the Isle of Man. During his confinement he began to refine his exercise techniques, combining everything that he had learnt from yoga, gymnastics, self-defence, weight training and martial arts, and practised his exercise programme with his fellow inmates.

He called this method of body conditioning '***Contrology***'. Joseph Pilates observed that if a body was misaligned or weak in a particular area, then muscles and joints would overcompensate in some way, often causing injuries. He continued to develop and refine his exercises, concentrating on physical remedies for postural misalignments.

After the war, Joseph Pilates returned to Germany. He taught self-defence to the Hamburg Military Police and the Army, and started working with Rudolf Laban (a dance artist and theorist), who introduced him to dance. In 1926, as a pacifist, Pilates became unhappy with the direction of German politics and decided to emigrate to America to join some of his relatives who were already living there.

On the ship travelling to America he met his future wife, Clara, who shared his passion for fitness. Arriving in the USA, together they set up a fitness studio in a building shared with the New York City Ballet. They trained actors, boxers, dancers and athletes to develop core strength, and

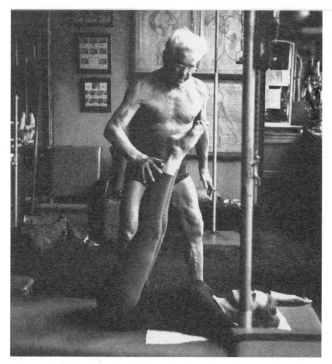

Joseph Pilates instructing a client and working her through an exercise routine in his studio in New York City (circa. 1961).

the 'Pilates method' became well known for rehabilitating those with injuries. Martha Graham, considered the mother of modern dance, was an early devotee, along with George Balanchine, the choreographer who transformed the American ballet world.

Joseph Pilates died in 1967 at the age of 83 of emphysema, which he contracted, it's believed, from a combination of factors – a fire in his studio the year before his death, and all the cigars he used to smoke.

By taking on apprentices and teaching them his programme of exercise, the Pilates method was passed on to others and continues to develop globally. Many of these 'Pilates Elders' as they were known went on to live long, healthy lives – a testament to the power of Pilates. The list is long and impressive. Clara, Joseph's wife, continued to teach after Joseph's death and lived to the grand age of 94. Romana Kryzanowska, a student of Joseph Pilates who took over his studio, died at the age of 90 in 2013. Mary Bowen and Lolita San Miguela are still alive and teaching.

The majority of health clubs and gyms hold mat Pilates sessions today. There are also many smaller independent classes held in church or village halls and private studios. I truly believe that by practising Pilates we too can live to a healthy and happy ripe old age.

> Contrology is complete coordination of body, mind and spirit designed to give you suppleness, natural grace and skill that will be unmistakably reflected in the way you walk, in the way you play, and in the way you work. You will develop muscular power with corresponding endurance, ability to perform arduous duties, to play strenuous games, to walk, run or travel for long distances without undue body fatigue or mental strain.
>
> Joseph Pilates, *Return to Life Through Contrology*

Chapter 2

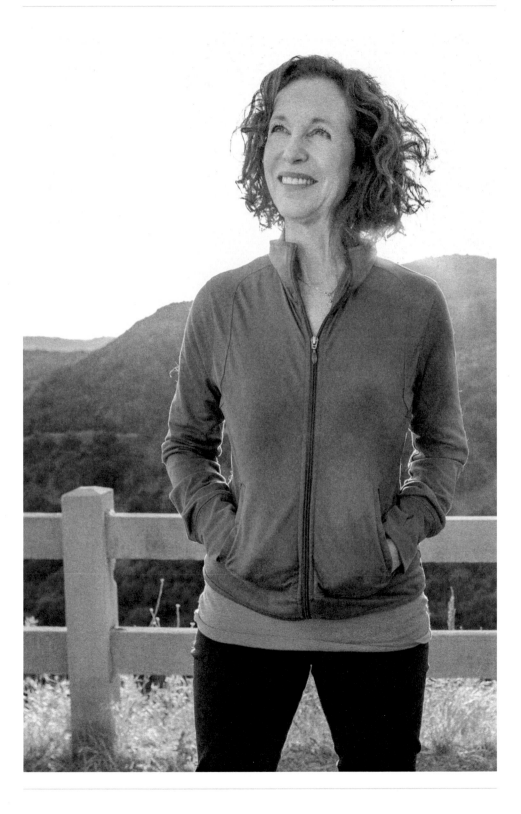

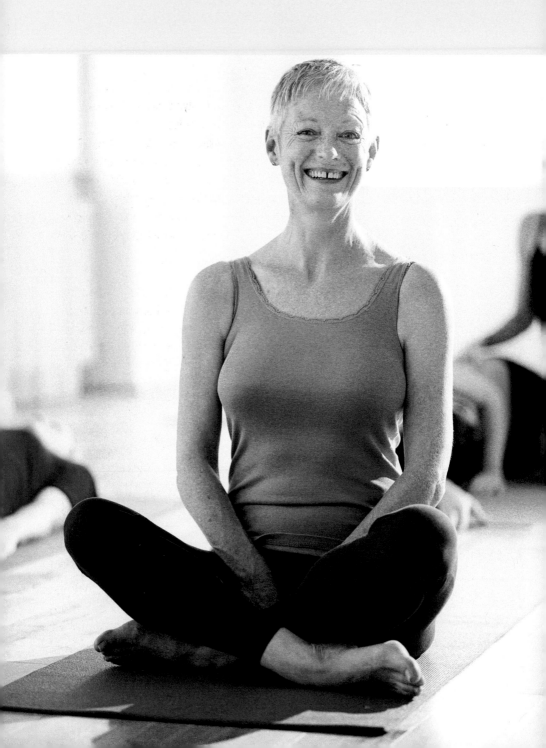

What Pilates can do for us as we age

Ageing successfully means learning how to make and maintain positive lifestyle changes to help us promote and remain in the best of health. Not just living longer, but better, and embracing later life rather than dreading it. Regular Pilates practice has the potential to enable this to happen. As we age, our bodies inevitably change. So it's vital we keep moving, not only to maintain our mobility and flexibility but also our confidence, our sense of self. But in order to keep comfortably mobile and to continue to do the things we've always done, we need to keep working on our strength, coordination and balance – and Pilates exercises are perfect for improving and maintaining these skills. We need to keep our torso strong (this is the middle part of our body) in order to support the movement of our arms and legs when we walk and generally move about in our daily lives. Although a cliché, 'use it or lose it' is true!

Think of your torso as the trunk and roots of a tree which needs to have a strong, solid foundation. If that trunk and its roots are weak, then the forces that the branches exert (your arms and legs) will uproot the tree, tip it over, and break it. The same goes for your body when you're moving about, stretching up to reach something in a high cupboard or bending over to pick up your shopping bags, or a child. As we age, sometimes these simple movements become more difficult.

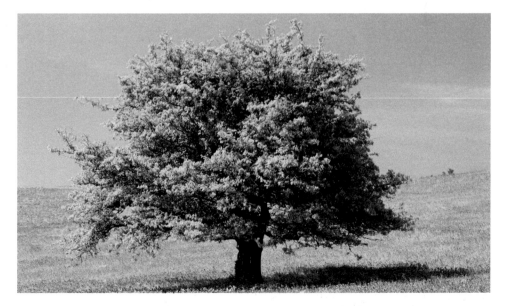

Pilates exercises are well known for improving core strength (the trunk and roots of the tree) and also posture and body alignment. An upright, lengthened body is a balanced, lighter body, which in turn will make you feel less tired and even, yes, dare I say it, younger. Especially when you're walking or jogging. Striding out with a lengthened spine is also psychologically uplifting — compare that to a round-shouldered stoop, head-down shuffle and the accompanying mood. Just try it.

> When all your muscles are properly developed, you will, as a matter of course, perform your work with minimum effort and maximum pleasure.
>
> Joseph Pilates

Core Muscles

Abdominal muscles

In Pilates we talk a lot about the 'core' or the 'powerhouse', as the abdominal muscles, your tummy, are sometimes known. Your core is made up of a collection of different muscle groups: the abdominal muscles, specifically the deepest, corset-like one which is called the **transversus abdominis** muscle — I've shortened it to TVA, so when you see those initials, you know I'm talking about deep tummy muscles. It wraps around your middle between the lower ribs and the top of the pelvis. This works together with your pelvic floor muscles. I talk in more detail about the pelvic floor muscles later on in the book (page 35). Both these sets of muscles support the pelvis and spine by maintaining something called **intra-abdominal pressure** during any exertion, like walking for example, while allowing your limbs to move freely. If you suffer from back problems — and sometimes this can be something that creeps up on us as we age, especially lower backache, or if you've spent years being sedentary — it can often be because these muscles are weak (see **lumbar spine**, page 30).

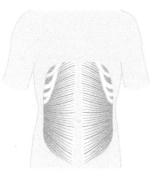

The transversus abdominis — this deep corset-like muscle wraps around our middle and works with the pelvic floor muscles to support the pelvis and spine — it's the one we need to engage when performing the exercises.

At the side of your tummy muscles are your internal and external oblique muscles — these are your waist muscles. On top of the deep TVA sits the more superficial **rectus abdominis** muscle, the 'six pack' — and yes, it's still possible to develop one as we grow older, it's really never too late! But it's the TVA that we are most interested in engaging and focusing on when performing Pilates exercises.

Glutes

Your **glutes** are your **gluteals**, or your buttock muscles. They are also important core muscles — they need to be strong for you to walk efficiently and climb stairs, or even better, climb those hills and mountains. You've heard the expression 'buns of steel' — so let's get some! If you have any back problems, you might have been told by your physiotherapist or osteopath during their examination that your glutes aren't 'firing'. This is a

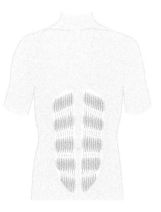

The rectus abdominis — our potential 'six pack'! It's never too late...

good example of a muscle imbalance. If your glutes aren't doing their job, which is to stabilize your pelvis, the muscles at the back of your thighs, your *hamstrings*, take over the job. You'll start to suffer from tight hamstrings and later, a tight or achy lower back can occur. See the Shoulder Bridge exercise (page 146) which is a wonderful glute-strengthening and back-mobilizing exercise. It will put you in touch with those buttock muscles in a way you never thought possible.

Back muscles

A set of important back muscles, the multifidus and erector spinae are also part of the core. The multifidus works with the TVA and pelvic floor muscles to stabilize the pelvis and lower back. The erector spinae extends (bends backwards) and laterally flexes the spine (side-to-side movement); it keeps the back upright and therefore plays a big part in our posture.

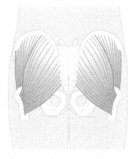

The glutes – buttock muscles that need to be strong to keep us walking efficiently, and climbing stairs and hills with ease.

All Pilates exercises work to strengthen and mobilize these really important core muscles. These are the main stabilizers of the torso and lower limbs. They keep the trunk upright and strong and we need them to function well so that we can move, walk, jog, climb, dance, ride horses or play tennis, reach high, reach low, pick up grandchildren and walk our dogs comfortably, while remaining injury and niggle-free. You'll find lots of back-strengthening and lengthening exercises in this book.

Balance

In order to balance well, you have to develop balance, or ***proprioception*** (the ability to sense the position, location and orientation of your limbs in space). This skill doesn't just happen by magic, and unfortunately, as we age we begin to lose our ability to balance, which makes us more susceptible to falls and injuries which could otherwise be prevented. So it is absolutely essential that we keep practising it, every day if possible, and I suggest ways of doing this in Chapter 8.

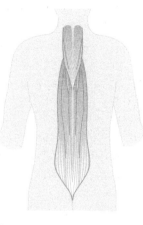

The erector spineae – extends and straightens the back, stabilizing the torso and enables side-to-side movement. It plays a big part in our posture.

Coordination

When we move about, walk or jog, we need to coordinate our arm and leg movements and be conscious of our intentions, sometimes referred to as *kinaesthetic sensing* (the ability to feel movements of the limbs and body). Remember the 'rub your tummy and pat your head' game? That's coordination. And once again it's a skill that tends to diminish in later life, which again has implications for injuries and falls, that end up making us

The Pilates method teaches you to be in control of your body and not at its mercy.

Joseph Pilates

feel elderly and frail, but could otherwise have been prevented. If we work at it, we can retain and improve our coordination skills.

So you can see how important good coordination and balance is for us as we get older. Many of the mat Pilates exercises in this book will challenge and improve your balance and coordination skills, while they also work on your core strength.

Breathing

Pilates breathing will help to strengthen your diaphragm and improve posture – the more upright and open your chest is, the easier it is to breathe and the better you will feel. When we become physically or mentally tired we tend to collapse from our centre. We become round-shouldered shufflers as we look down at the ground – not an attractive look! This curved posture restricts the movement of the diaphragm and lungs.

Good lung capacity means that when you move about you are able to transfer maximum oxygen into your body and muscles in order to optimize whatever activity you are doing. You need to be able to use your lungs fully and expand your rib cage comfortably, utilizing the diaphragm to power that breathing.

> If your spine is inflexibly stiff at 30, you are old. If it is completely flexible at 60, you are young.
>
> Joseph Pilates

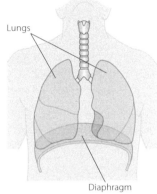

Lungs

Diaphragm

The diaphragm – a major breathing muscle. By practising the Pilates breathing, improving posture and strengthening your diaphragm, you'll feel more energized.

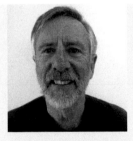

CASE STUDY

Alastair Hatchett
Age: 70
Practised Pilates for: 20 years
Favourite exercise: The Hundred (page 141)

'In my 40s I experienced occasional back pain. I read that Pilates was a good way of exercising to prevent back problems through building core strength, and since beginning my practice I've rarely had any problems over the past 20 years. My general health has also been good. I've developed arthritis in the past ten years and Pilates has helped combat this through stretching and maintaining muscle strength. I walk at least 6km every day, despite osteoarthritis in one foot, and in the past year I have started swimming twice a week. I cycle a bit. Pilates has helped me to maintain flexibility and counters sore knees, feet and hips. I think anyone who goes to the gym, runs or plays football or lifts small children regularly should start practising Pilates to maintain health and strength as they get older.'

Practising Pilates breathing, improving posture and strengthening the diaphragm will not only enhance your movement and chosen activities but also your general everyday wellbeing. You'll feel more energized because your body is receiving more oxygen, and your overall demeanour will be one of energy and positivity – which in turn will make you feel younger.

Stretching

As we age we tend to get a little stiffer and less flexible. There is a lot of conflicting research out there about how important stretching actually is in our day-to-day life, but I believe it is vital. If the muscles remain shortened, not stretched, which they do if you sit all day and don't move much, they become tight and weak, and niggles develop, and injury can follow.

Pilates improves flexibility by constantly lengthening the muscles during the exercises. In order that we retain full, comfortable mobility in whatever activity we choose to do, or in our day-to-day living, we need our muscles to be long.

Posture

Pilates improves overall posture, and Chapter 5 is dedicated to postural alignment because it is such an important part of *Pilates for Living*. There are so many elements of posture to consider.

Good posture – how you hold your body against gravity when moving about or walking – is vital in order that you can move efficiently, with greater ease and with far less stress on the body. When your posture is good, there is literally less strain on the joints and bones because they are held in correct alignment. Muscles will remain lengthened and strong. Your legs and arms will be free to work hard at propelling you comfortably forwards as you walk up that hill or jog along the sea front. How often do we see older people depicted as frail, hunchbacked shufflers? We need to end that image right now.

Before any real benefit can be derived from physical exercises, one must first learn how to breathe properly. Our very life depends on it.

Joseph Pilates

Good posture can be successfully acquired only when the entire mechanism of the body is under perfect control. Graceful carriage follows as a matter of course.

Joseph Pilates

Chapter 3

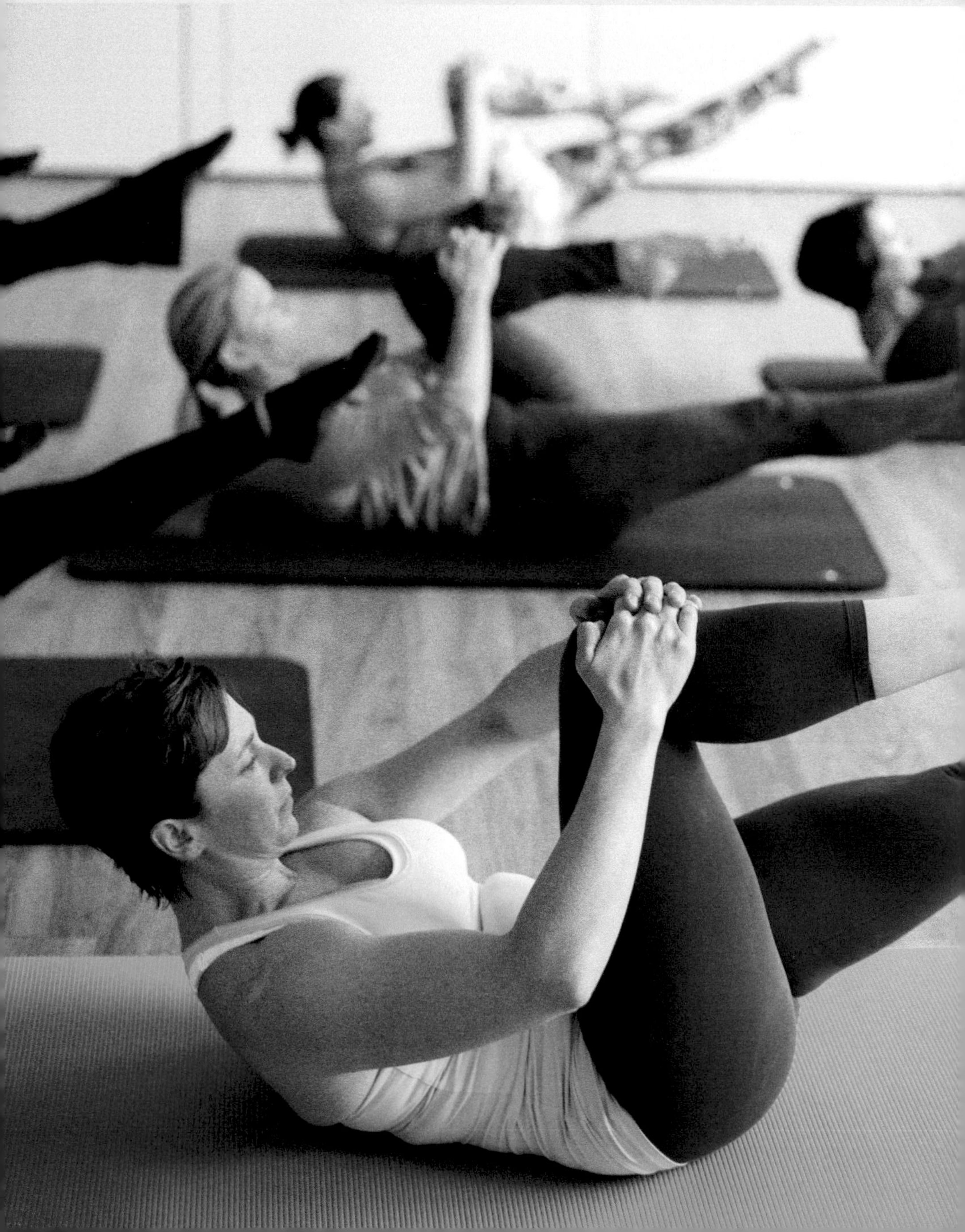

What is Pilates?
The Pilates principles

Joseph Pilates maintained that by following his exercise programme you would gain total control of your body. Losing control can be something we fear on lots of levels as we age. Pilates makes us stronger and more able, which gives us confidence and in turn keeps us motivated to live more actively in our later years. In addition, Joseph Pilates devised specific principles that he believed were necessary to accompany each of his exercises. Over the years, different schools of Pilates have adapted these principles or added a variety of others to the list, but all are still respectful of, and relevant to, the Pilates method.

The following Pilates principles are worth keeping in the forefront of your mind and applying when performing the exercises in this book. They can also, of course, be applied to our lives in general at whatever stage of life we're at.

Concentration

Our ability to concentrate can change as we get older, but by performing the exercises in this book and focusing on practising concentration we can improve this skill. Being able to apply oneself wholly to the task in hand and block out any distractions isn't easy at the best of times in our frenetic world. Once you are familiar with the exercises in this book, you will find it easier to focus fully on each movement, allowing them to become flowing and connected. Try not to let your mind wander, ignore your 'to do' list, switch off your phone and instead begin to feel the connection between concentrating your mind and the movements of your body.

Eventually, with practice, the movement patterns will become second nature to you. Your concentration will improve and you'll begin to notice changes in the way you move and feel.

This is a form of mindfulness — by performing the exercises, being at one with the moment, observing how it feels and paying full attention to your body and its response.

> Concentrate on the correct movements each time you exercise, lest you do them improperly.
>
> Joseph Pilates

Breathing

Quite simply, we need to breathe to live. But how well do we actually breathe? In Pilates *lateral thoracic breathing* (page 30) helps the exercise to flow, aids concentration and allows the body to relax into the movement. If you're a breath-holder when you exercise, you're not allowing your muscles to receive the oxygen that they need, which stresses the body and makes the movements more difficult. So it's worth trying to master the correct breathing technique at the same time as you learn the exercises. Pilates breathing is integral to the correct execution of the exercises and will strengthen your diaphragm, which in turn will increase your everyday stamina.

> Breathing is the first act of life, and the last.
>
> Joseph Pilates

Centring

'Core stability' is a modern term, not coined by Joseph Pilates. However, he referred to the core as the 'powerhouse' of the body. All Pilates exercises come from this strong centre. By activating the TVA and pelvic floor muscles, we increase the overall strength and stability of the torso. Staying centred also refers to the mind: concentrating on the movement, being in the moment and focusing on what is happening in and to your body.

Alignment

Joseph Pilates called this 'precision': placing your muscles and joints in the correct position when performing the exercises. To read more about the *Neutral Spine*, see page 32. When the body is aligned from head to toe it's in its strongest position, where your muscles and joints can function optimally in whatever activity you choose to perform, whether it's walking, dancing, bowling, playing golf, horse riding or jogging. Pilates teaches you optimum alignment through its emphasis on improving posture, and you'll be checking your alignment before and during every exercise. Postural alignment is something you can start thinking about and apply immediately once you understand the process. When you next go out for a walk you'll be thinking about it and feeling the difference.

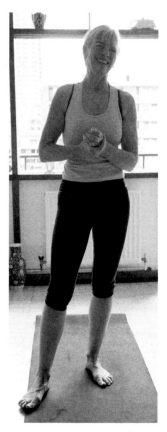

Relaxation

Stay aware and recognize any tightness or tension that occurs in your body as you perform the exercises. Shoulders can rise up around the ears without you even realizing it, fists can be clenched and jaws locked. I see this all the time in my Pilates classes. Dealing with any tensions in the body means that eventually they will disappear, making it easier to execute the movements required. When you fully relax your body you will be slowing your heart rate down, which in turn will relieve stress. If you have high blood pressure, it will be beneficial to learn to fully relax. It will also improve your sleep (page 198).

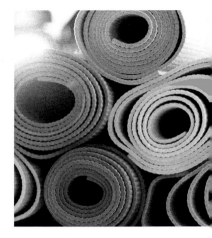

Flow

All the movements in Pilates are designed to flow smoothly and gently into each other as you lengthen and strengthen your muscles. When you first begin practising Pilates you might find that the movements can be a bit jerky or rigid as you get used to what you need to do. Or you might find you need to rest between each action, which is absolutely fine. Admittedly there's a lot to think about, but be patient and over time this will change. Once again, be aware of what your body is doing, stay connected to what's happening and you'll find the flow will come naturally. And once you've mastered the breathing it will make all the difference to how you produce flowing movements.

Stamina

By challenging your stability and regularly working your muscles when practising Pilates exercises, as you increase the repetitions and move on to more challenging exercises, you will be building strength and stamina. Including Pilates in your weekly routine will pay dividends to how you feel. And of course, this transfers to your everyday activities: the stronger you become, the more you'll build resistance to any niggles that might be lurking and be able to comfortably and safely sustain whatever it is you choose to do as you grow older.

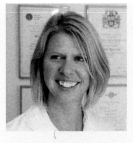

PROFESSIONAL ADVICE

Osteopath, Jane Kaushal says:

'The reason why it is important to increase or maintain bone mass in older age is to prevent osteoporosis-related fractures. In order to prevent reduction in bone mass it is helpful to "overload" the bones with jumping-type activities or heavy weight training. Pilates practice would need to be very vigorous to "tick these boxes". However, Pilates can have an even more important impact on prevention of osteoporosis-related fractures because it provides significant benefits to balance, postural stability, muscle strength and flexibility. This all helps with fall prevention. While being more active improves health in numerous ways, it can also mean that you are more likely to fall. This is not so likely to be the case if you regularly practise Pilates.'

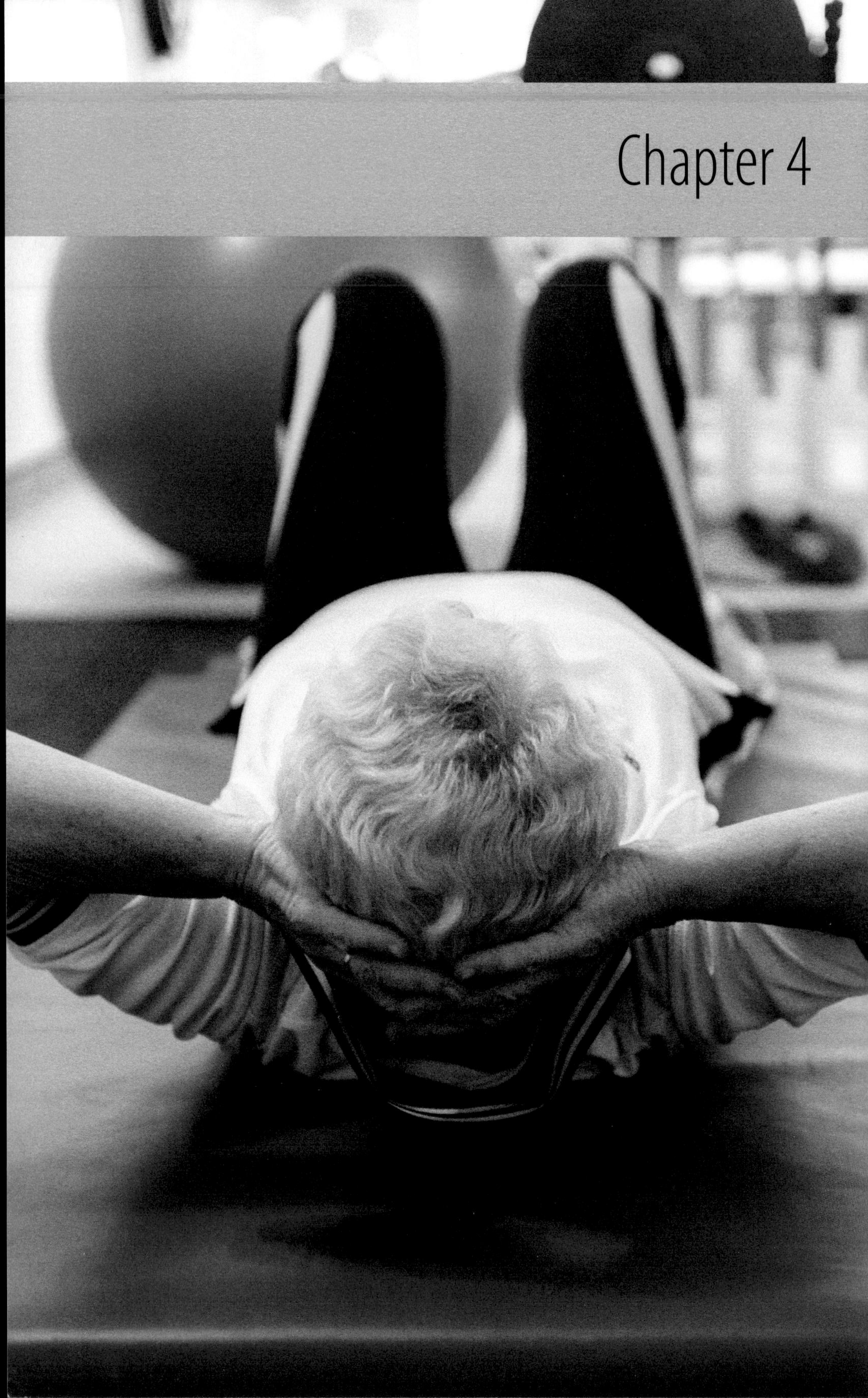

Chapter 4

Equipment

Before we go any further it's a good idea to make sure you have everything you need at hand to practise the exercises comfortably and successfully. Pilates, in general, just requires a mat. Having said that, I have included some extra equipment in some of the more advanced exercises to make them more challenging. It's up to you whether you choose to use these in your weekly programme or not. Before you start it's a good idea to get yourself prepared. Wear comfortable clothes in which you can move around freely – loose fitting T-shirt and leggings or tracksuit bottoms are good – and make sure you have enough space around you. Ideally, all exercises should be performed in bare feet or socks.

- **A Pilates or yoga mat** makes for a more comfortable experience. You will need some cushioning, especially when lying on your front or side, rolling or if you have had a hip or knee replacement. There are different types of mats on the market, but I would suggest a thicker one so that your spine and joints are better protected. If you practise your Pilates on a hard rather than carpeted floor, you will need to make sure you have a mat that won't slip and that your hands and feet can grip on to as well.

- **A small, firm foam block** ($20 \times 15 \times 2$cm) is useful, or you can use a rolled-up towel or small cushion to put under your head, so that your neck and spine stay aligned. Everyone's posture is different, so you will need to experiment with this. If you find that your head tilts back, sending your chin into the air when lying down flat with nothing supporting your head, place the block underneath to bring your neck into alignment. If, however, the opposite happens and your chin comes forwards on to your chest when you place your head on the block, don't use one. Think about placement – are your neck and spine aligned? And then adjust accordingly.

- **Dyna-Bands™ or yoga straps** for stretching and hip circles are cheap and very versatile pieces of kit.

- **Foot roller or foot massage ball** (a tennis ball is also fine) are great for tired feet.

- **Small hand weights** are an excellent addition but are, of course, optional. In some of the exercise progressions I make suggestions about when you might like to use light hand weights. In my classes we use soft ball-shaped weights which are safer than the hard ones for these type of exercises. Or you can make your own by filling small plastic water bottles with sand or water.

- **Ankle weights** – again, these are optional and in some of the Side Series advanced exercises I have suggested you might want to use them to increase the challenge (pages 110–119).

Note: it's important that you can execute the exercises in a flowing, smooth and comfortable fashion, keeping correct alignment throughout, before adding in any weights. Choose ankle and hand weights that weigh 0.5kg or 1kg. As your strength improves you can include heavier weights. Experiment to see what works for you.

1) Hand weights
2) Head blocks
3) Massage roller
4) Dyna-Band™
5) Mat
6) Massage balls
7) Ankle weights
8) Soft, thick block

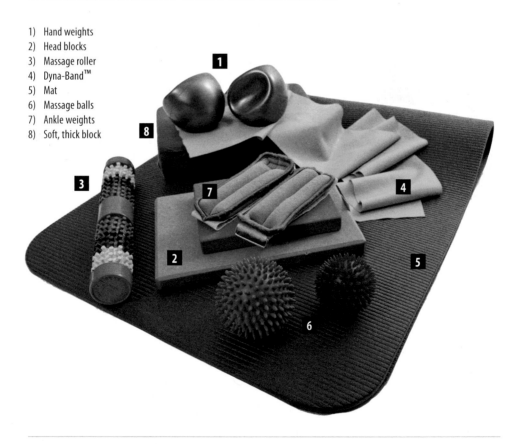

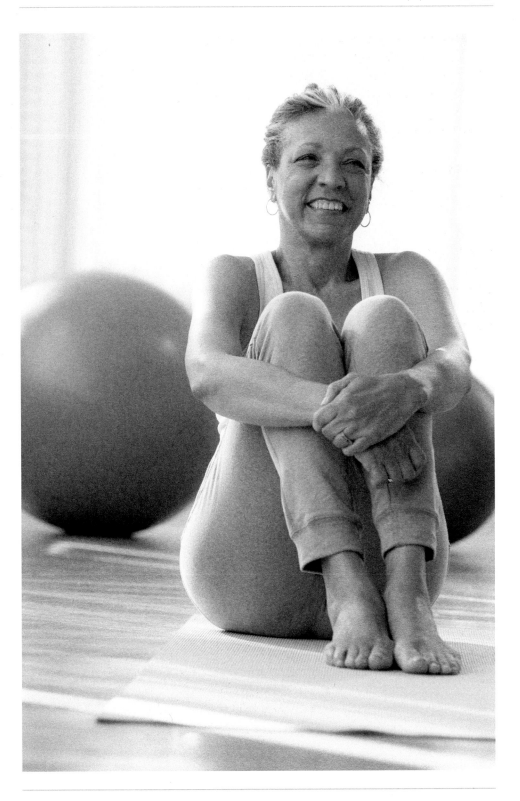

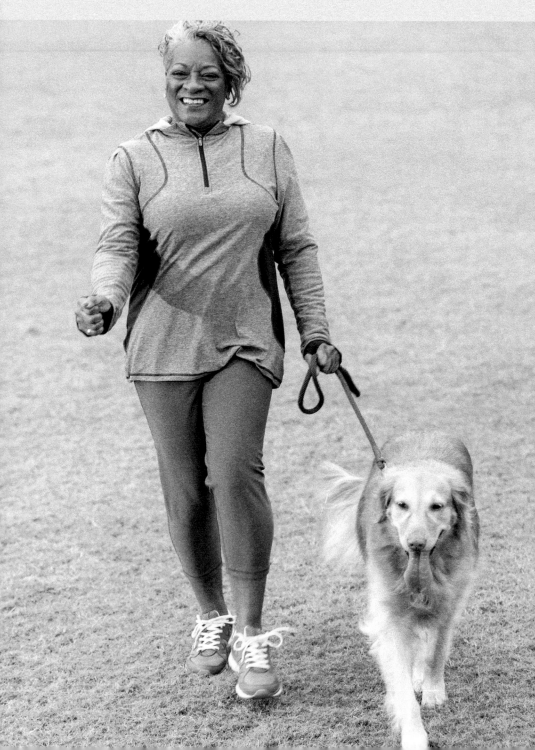

Chapter 5

Postural alignment for living

When you're next out walking, do a bit of people watching. Sit on a park bench and watch the world go by. Take a look at all the different sorts of postures there are. Some people walk along looking as if the weight of the world is carried upon their shoulders, while others stick out their chins and chests as if in a perpetual rush.

Do you look at the path or your feet (or your phone), maybe deep in thought, as you walk? Or do you lift your head up and look forwards towards the horizon? Do you shuffle? Or lift up your feet? What are your arms doing? Are your fists clenched? I think you can tell a lot about someone's personality, mood and lifestyle by their posture.

If you sit in front of a computer all day, then maybe you have a tendency to have rounded shoulders and you'll probably have tight *hip flexors* as well – hip flexors help lift your legs as you walk. Or maybe your knees will ache. If you cross your legs; if your computer isn't at eye level; if you feel unhappy or in pain; if you wear high heels; walk with a limp – everything can affect your posture. In addition, anxieties can turn into tension, and unresolved emotions can manifest themselves in stress-related niggles or injuries. So it's not surprising that we end up with a body that compensates and then starts to complain as the years progress.

Posture can also affect our wellbeing; standing upright, lengthening through the spine with an open chest and relaxed shoulders immediately feels better than being slouched and scrunched up in a defeated, collapsed stance.

As we age our posture can change a lot, so it's important to start looking after it and become body-aware as early as possible. With good posture, all your vital organs will be held in the right place, everything will function well and you will move so much more easily and freely as you go about your everyday life and activities. Pilates will start sorting it out right away.

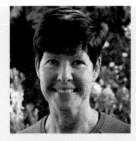

CASE STUDY

Andrea Holmes
Age: 54
Practised Pilates for: 4 years
Favourite exercise: Roll Up with Spinal Stretch (page 164)

'I took up Pilates because I wanted to try a different sort of exercise and I became hooked! I love stretching and want to remain flexible as I age – it's also really good for my back and shoulders which sometimes ache. It loosens them up. My posture has improved and I feel stronger – I really notice that I tend to stiffen up if I don't practise Pilates and find it's not as easy to move, bend or pick things up like my grandchild!'

The Spine

When we move, whether fast or slow, walking or jogging, our bodies are supported by the spine. It keeps us upright and carries the weight of our head, torso and arms. Good, upright walking, and learning to keep the spine in its strongest, safest position with the least stress placed on discs and ligaments, will make all the difference to your body and how you feel.

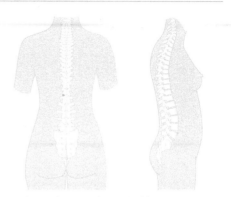

A normal spine – what we should all aspire to.

Lumbar spine

This is your lower back, and where most people find they get discomfort as they age. If your abdominal muscles have become weakened over time, then it's possible they are not doing their job of keeping this part of your back protected. If the TVA, which acts as a corset, wrapping itself around your middle (page 16), is not 'laced up properly', it can allow the abdominal muscles to fall forwards – think beer belly! So strengthening the abdominal muscles and 'lacing up your corset' is vital for a healthy lower back.

Lordosis is the name given to an excessive curvature or arch of the lower back. Flat back posture is where there is little mobility in the lower back. Both these conditions can develop over the years through muscular imbalances caused by lifestyle choices and/or genetic disposition.

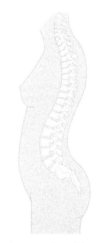

A lordotic spine – curvature of the lower back.

Thoracic spine

This is the mid-upper back that can morph into a round-shouldered hunch. Many of the exercises in this book talk about strengthening or mobilising the *thoracic spine*. However, in reality it's not designed to be a very mobile part of the back as it has to be stable to house our vital organs: the heart and lungs. This part of our back supports the chest and rib cage as we breathe in and out. It also provides added support to our heads – so if alignment isn't quite right, then this part of our back and the areas it supports will suffer.

Kyphosis is a condition in which the upper back curves excessively and the shoulders are rounded. If you work in an office and sit at a desk all day, or if you are very tall, you might be familiar with this hunched, round-shouldered posture. Not something we want to encourage as we age.

Swayback posture can be recognised by the increased curvature of the thoracic spine (kyphosis), as well as a backward tilt of the pelvis, creating a lordosis in the lower lumbar spine so it looks flat, pushing the hips forward.

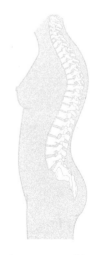

A kyphotic spine – curvature of the mid/upper back.

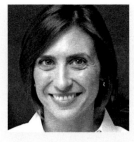

PROFESSIONAL ADVICE

GP and Pilates advocate Dr Helen Kennedy, who has a special interest in women's health, says:

'Exercise is clearly important as we age for both physical and mental benefits. Women need to fight the effects of oestrogen deficiency and maintain muscle strength and bulk as well as flexibility to reduce unwanted symptoms. Weight-bearing exercise is important for bone health, along with an adequate intake of calcium and vitamin D, but for a more holistic approach, consideration should also be given to muscle toning – and Pilates is an ideal way to do this. It can be practised at different levels of intensity to suit different abilities, and built up at a pace to suit the individual. The benefits of exercise on mental wellbeing are also well documented. As we get older, and particularly after the menopause, it is normal for us to gain weight and oestrogen deficiency causes a redistribution of body fat to around the abdomen, giving us more of an apple shape. Practising Pilates can help to maintain a healthy weight and improve posture, both of which can lead to an improvement in body shape, and consequently self-confidence. Apart from the satisfaction in knowing that you are being healthy, exercise releases "happy hormones" in the same way that antidepressant medication can, and is an important part of managing low mood and anxiety which can also be more common at this time of life.'

Over time, Pilates exercises will encourage awareness to help you improve and go some way to correcting these postural imbalances. In turn this will have a positive effect on your whole demeanour. But the first thing you need to do is familiarize yourself with your own posture, so that you can start improving it. Maybe you've never thought about how you stand, sit or walk – so take your time and have a good look. As you progress through the exercises and practise regularly, you will notice the difference that Pilates has made.

Alignment is everything. Throughout all the exercises in this book we are working on postural alignment, whether lying on your front, back, side or standing.

The following information is essential to be able to understand the Pilates exercises. You may need to keep referring back. Please read through the whole section to begin with, take a look at the pictures and then have a practise: not only will your posture start to improve right away, but the exercises will be easier to execute. It might help to have someone read out the following information to you when you perform the movements for the first time.

Neutral Spine

All Pilates exercises start from Neutral Spine or sometimes imprinted spine (page 37). Neutral Spine is a good, strong, healthy position and what we need to be aiming for.

Neutral Spine when lying down

This is the position in which your spine and pelvis are aligned and arranged in their strongest position in their natural curves, with the least amount of stress placed on the discs and ligaments.

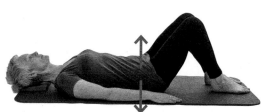

- To familiarize yourself with this position, lie on your back, bend your knees and place your feet parallel and in line with your hips.
- Take your arms down by your sides.
- Now tilt your pelvis backwards and forwards comfortably a few times, producing a pronounced arch under your lower back, then flattening your spine down on to the floor.
- These are exaggerated moves; Neutral Spine is the middle position between the two.
- This position should be relaxed, not forced and feel natural.

Neutral Spine when standing up

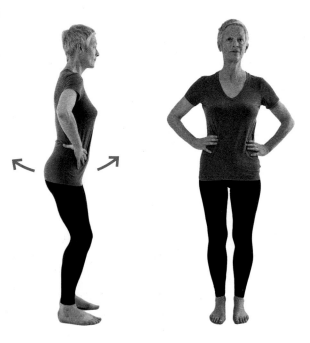

- Stand tall, spine lengthened, with your feet in line with your hips.
- Place your hands on your hips.
- Rock your pelvis backwards and forwards – feel the movement under your hands.
- Imagine your pelvis is a bowl of water.
- When you tilt your pelvis forwards, the water from the bowl spills out the front.
- When you tilt your pelvis backwards the water from the bowl spills out the back.
- Bring the pelvis/bowl to the centre position where the water stays level and doesn't spill. That's Neutral Spine.

Throughout the exercises in this book I suggest 'pelvic tilts' as a way of finding your Neutral Spine – this is the action of moving your pelvis backwards and forwards, as described. It's also a great, simple exercise for a tight achy back after a walk, a lengthy gardening spree or if you've been sitting for too long.

Standing Tall

During the warm-up sequence to the Pilates exercises it's important to take some time to learn how to stand tall and remain centred. This will transfer to all your movements in everyday life. If you can stand in front of a long mirror when you do the warm-up, it will give you a better idea of your posture, what needs to happen to improve it and what good posture looks like. If you're feeling a little daunted by the exercises, stick with the warm-up for a while until you're happy and confident with the movements, then progress by having a go at the Starter Pack exercises (page 68) until you feel ready to begin the main exercises in *Pilates for Living*.

Take a good look at how you stand:
- Does your head tilt a little to one side?
- Are your shoulders level or is one higher than the other?
- Are your hips level?
- Is your weight evenly distributed between your feet or are you leaning slightly?

Stand sideways and take a look at your lower back:
- Does it arch? (See lumbar spine, page 30)

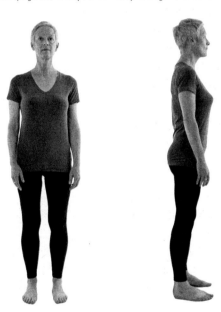

Look at the middle of your back:
- Is it rounded? (See thoracic spine, page 30)
- Does your chin jut out?
- Do you have rounded shoulders?
- Is your chest elevated in a military stance?

Experts sometimes use what's called a 'plumb line' when taking a look at posture from the side. This is the line of gravity that runs vertically from your ear lobe down to the outside of your ankle bone.
- Once you have become familiar with your own postural alignment, turn back to face the mirror.
- Place your feet directly below your hips and make sure that they are facing forwards – not turned out at 'ten-to-two' or 'toe to toe'. Your weight should be evenly distributed.

- Notice whether your knees are above your ankles – sometimes knees come together a little; if yours do, be aware of it and correct accordingly.
- Place your hips above your knees.
- Relax your arms by your sides.
- Lengthen through your spine, imagining you have a big bunch of helium balloons attached to the top of your head lifting you upwards – notice how you immediately grow taller and feel lighter.
- Keep this lengthening in your spine. Don't forget to lengthen your neck too.
- Keep your chin parallel to the floor and your gaze focused straight ahead.
- Relax your shoulders.
- Relax your jaw.
- Notice the changes and how different you feel.

> Standing also is very important and should be practised at all times until it is mastered … never slouch, as doing so compresses the lungs, overcrowds other vital organs, rounds the back and throws off the balance.
>
> Joseph Pilates

Engaging Your Muscles

When you perform the Pilates exercises in this book you will need to engage your deep abdominal muscles (TVA) and your pelvic floor muscles before you move. When you first start practising Pilates it can be hard to do both at the same time, so although in the exercises I mention both, choose one – take your time to experiment and get to know how each contraction feels and what difference they make to the execution of the exercises.

The following visualization and exercise will demonstrate how to do this, and once again it's something that you can start practising straight away: in the supermarket queue, at the bus stop, walking the dog, in the kitchen while you're cooking – anywhere really!

Abdominal muscles
- Imagine you have a big belt wrapped around your waist. The belt has 10 notches.
- Visualize pulling the belt to the 10th notch so that your abdomen is pulled right in as far as it will go – not very comfortable or very realistic!
- Relax.
- Now pull the imaginary belt halfway to the 5th notch so it is a little more comfortable for your abdominal muscles.
- Relax.
- Now pull the imaginary belt to the 3rd notch.
- Generally this is where you want to be pulling your abdominal muscles in to each time you perform an exercise: the 3rd notch on your imaginary belt.

However, you might find that you'll have to increase to the 5th notch on your imaginary belt when performing some of the more advanced exercises.

When you are pulling your TVA in, you are supporting and stabilizing your spine, immediately making your torso stronger. Try doing this when you're walking too, keeping those abdominal muscles activated for as long as possible. You will immediately feel a difference.

Pelvic floor muscles

Alongside the TVA, the pelvic floor muscles work to help stabilize and support the spine and pelvis by maintaining *intra-abdominal pressure* during any exertion. Walking or jogging increases this intra-abdominal pressure, so a weak pelvic floor can lead to all sorts of problems, for both men and women. As we age, due to loss of muscle mass and collagen depletion – and for women, pregnancy and childbirth is an obvious added factor – our pelvic floor muscles weaken, which can lead to urinary incontinence.

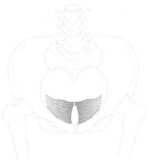

The pelvic floor muscles – these are important to activate and keep strong for lots of reasons as we age

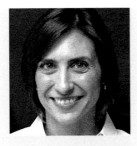

PROFESSIONAL ADVICE

GP and Pilates advocate Dr Helen Kennedy who has a special interest in women's health, describes the pelvic floor and talks about the benefits of pelvic floor exercises as we age:

'The pelvic floor is a sheet of muscle and connective tissue that spans the area underneath the pelvis, providing support to the pelvic organs including the bladder, bowel and, in women, the womb. If there is not adequate support it can lead to prolapse and also to stress incontinence, which is where leakage of urine occurs with coughing, sneezing, jumping, or any activity that leads to a rise in pressure in the abdomen.

As we age, it is common for the pelvic floor to weaken, often for a combination of reasons. Giving birth can cause problems later in life and make us more prone to prolapse and urinary incontinence. Even without a vaginal delivery, just the weight of carrying round a baby during pregnancy can weaken the pelvic floor. Another important factor can be the menopause, when we experience declining levels of oestrogen which is important in maintaining the quality and strength of muscle and connective tissue.

There is good evidence that pelvic floor exercises are beneficial in the management of urinary incontinence in women and are used as a first line of treatment before other options such as surgery are considered. Up to 70 per cent improvement can be seen in symptoms when exercises are done correctly and consistently. The exercises can also be helpful in improving symptoms of prolapse. Specialist physiotherapy may be offered to those with more severe problems, but having an awareness of your pelvic floor through practising Pilates will undoubtedly be beneficial. Strengthening and pulling up that muscle "sling" will lift the pelvic organs and keep them where they are meant to be and work best.'

Pilates exercises are an excellent way to strengthen the pelvic floor muscles to prevent urinary incontinence — so if yours are weak and you have problems as a result, these exercises will begin to fix it.

- To contract your pelvic floor muscles, the simplest way to describe it is to imagine stopping the flow of urine when you go for a wee. This applies to both men and women. Or imagine trying to stop breaking wind in public, by lifting up your back passage. It's an internal lift: there should be no external 'clenching'!
- Notice as you pull your pelvic floor muscles up how your TVA activates at the same time — proof, if you need it, that these two sets of muscles work together to support the spine and stabilize the pelvis.

Shoulder Stabilization

Maintaining shoulder stabilization during Pilates exercises is another important part of postural alignment. An awareness of what your shoulders are doing will help you to perform the exercises without them becoming tense and inadvertently ending up around your ears. If you suffer from tight shoulders, this will help relieve the tension.

- Lift both your shoulders right up to your ears.
- Soften them back and down — imagine your shoulder blades sliding down towards the back pockets of your trousers, keeping your neck long.
- Relax your shoulders completely, and then repeat a few more times, lifting up to your ears and then melting your shoulder blades down.

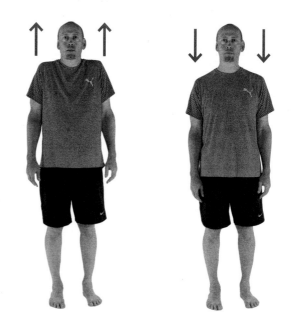

This is a great way to open out the chest and help the shoulders relax — something you can perform if you've been sitting hunched over your desk for a long time, or driving for hours.

Imprinting the Spine

You will only need to imprint your spine if you are unable to keep Neutral Spine when both your feet are lifted off the ground (see The Hundred, page 141). If finding Neutral Spine is a challenge and your abdominal muscles don't feel strong enough to support your spine, then it can be advisable to adopt this position before you move your legs off the mat and into *Table Top* position.

- Lie on your back, knees bent with your feet in line with your hips.
- Engage your abdominal muscles and sink your back very gently down into the floor as if 'imprinting' it on the mat.

- Raise one leg up into Table Top – this is when your knee is placed above your hip and your shin is parallel to the ceiling.

- Raise the other leg up into Table Top to join it.

This 'imprinting' position is all about ensuring that your back is in a safe position when your legs are raised if you're unable to sustain Neutral Spine. if you have a serious back problem, please consult your medical practitioner to check that this position is safe for your paritcular condition.

Chapter 6

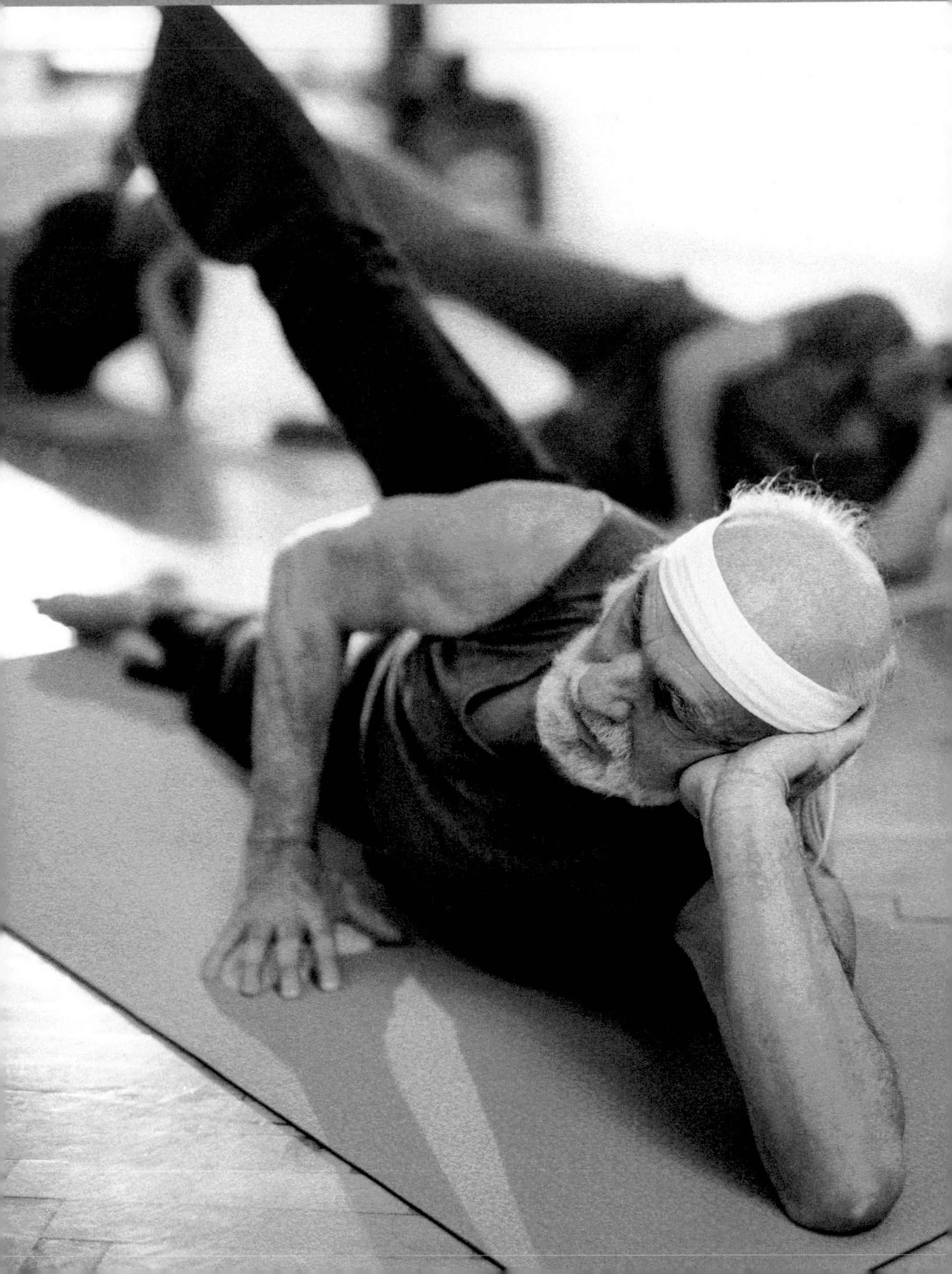

Breathing

Pilates Breathing

Pilates breathing is known as '*lateral thoracic breathing*'.

- Stand tall and lengthen through your spine.
- Breathe in deeply, through your nose, into your rib cage, and then slowly breathe out through your mouth.

The reason we do this lateral thoracic breathing into the rib cage and not into the abdominal cavity is so that you can activate your tummy muscles at the same time as breathing – if you were belly breathing it would be quite challenging to pull the abdominal muscles in.

- Place your hands either side of your torso on your rib cage.
- Breathe in through the nose and feel how the rib cage expands underneath your hands.
- Breathe out slowly through your mouth and allow your rib cage to relax.
- Try not to let your shoulders rise up as you breathe.
- Practise this breathing a few times.

Pilates breathing helps the exercises to flow, strengthens your diaphragm and encourages you to relax the body. For some people this is the hardest part of practising Pilates, so take your time if you find the lateral thoracic breathing challenging. Try it out every now and again, and slowly you will find yourself getting into the rhythm of it. Whatever happens, just remember to breathe when you perform the exercises – don't hold your breath!

Lateral thoracic breathing, the breathing we adopt in Pilates, will strengthen your diaphragm, which does 80 per cent of the breathing work. We can't make our lungs any bigger but we can improve our posture to help those lungs and our diaphragms function more efficiently, which in turn will improve our overall stamina and how we feel as we grow older.

Chapter 7

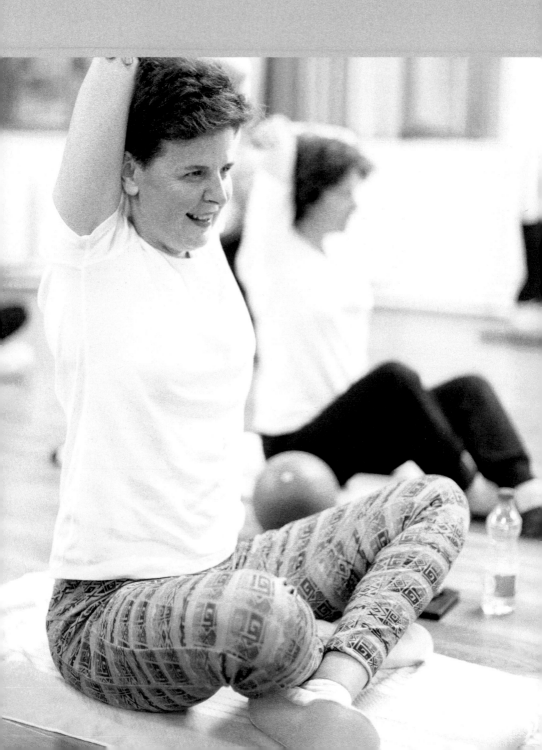

Gentle warm-up exercises for everyone

Before you start, a note on hip and knee replacements, arthritis and breast surgery. Obviously there are many other conditions and problems which could be mentioned here but, along with general back problems, these are the ones I most often see in my classes.

Pilates is a wonderful way to restore your energy post-illness, or post-operatively, and regain your strength, mobility, flexibility and balance. But please do take professional advice if you're in any doubt at all about the suitability of the movements you're performing in relation to any problem you may have. Many physiotherapists, sports therapists, osteopaths, chiropractors and GPs recommend Pilates but there may be some moves that are contraindicated as a result of your condition – **please make sure that if you're under the care of any of the above practitioners, you take their advice and work with them. They will tell you what you can and can't do and give you the right advice.**

General back problems

Pilates improves core strength and so in many cases can alleviate back problems, but it is important that you take it easy and read the instructions fully before attempting any of the exercises. In the following chapters you will read many case studies from people with back problems who have found that Pilates has relieved them of discomfort and given them a new lease of life. And, as I've already stated, please take advice from a medical professional before attempting the exercises. There is more on posture and back problems in Chapter 5.

Hip replacement

Pilates is an excellent way to strengthen and recover after a hip replacement. The exercises can restore your natural range of movement and improve your posture. Pre-operatively your postural alignment might have been altered due to pain and restricted movement. All this can be rectified and correct movement patterns and strength restored. However, it is important to avoid hip flexion past 90 degrees – this means not bending your knee up too high or hip too far. And no crossing your legs or taking

> I started Pilates 6 months after I broke my shoulder. Without a doubt it improved the movement, felt stronger and was less stiff. It gave me more confidence to use my arm and shoulder.
>
> Hilary Bentley (you can read Hilary's full case study on page 135).

your leg across the centre of your body. Your physiotherapist will be able to advise you on when you can begin practising Pilates and which exercises are appropriate for you to perform.

Knee replacement

Pilates exercises will help improve the strength of the muscles surrounding the knee, particularly the thigh muscles and help you regain full range of movement to your knee. Pre-operatively you might have been limping and your movement limited, so give your body time to readjust. The balance, core strengthening and foot and ankle mobility exercises will all help you get back to normal. However, avoid any of the kneeling exercises and certainly in the early stages of rehab. The Shoulder Bridge (page 146) should be avoided.

Arthritis

I see many clients with arthritis in my classes. Pilates is a wonderful form of exercise for anyone suffering from this condition. The exercises are low-impact, gentle and can help reduce pain, increasing range of movement in stiff joints while improving strength and flexibility. It may be the last thing you feel like doing but I promise once you get going you'll find yourself feeling so much better and more able. Arthritis UK has lots of information on exercise hints and tips and mentions Pilates. See www.arthritisresearchuk.org for more information.

Ann Dunn has had two knees and one hip replaced:

The main benefit of doing Pilates when suffering from arthritis is keeping the body moving but most importantly strengthening the muscles supporting the joints. Strengthening the muscles can stave off an early operation – it also means that the joints are less painful. The physio said I made a good movement recovery because my muscles were strong and I did the exercises recommended. I also think doing Pilates puts you in the right frame of mind for doing the post-op exercises.

(You can read Ann's full case study on page 116).

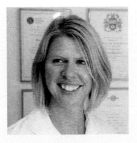

PROFESSIONAL ADVICE

Osteopath Jane Kaushal says:

'We all have signs of wear and tear in our joints past the age of 25. This will continue through the rest of our lives – resistance is futile! But numerous studies show that a person's symptoms do not have a direct correlation to their scan findings. You can have two people with similar hip X-ray findings, and one is in a lot of pain and the other is doing much better. The reason for this difference is the "context" of that hip and the health of the muscles, and other joints that affect the area. If you keep strong and flexible with good balance, by practising Pilates regularly, you are more likely to cope well with wear and tear and be able to do what you want to do, without pain, for longer.'

Breast surgery

After breast surgery, arm and shoulder movement can be restricted and sometimes a tightness felt in the armpit and chest. Practising Pilates, especially the arm and shoulder mobility exercises (page 130–137), can help you regain movement so that you can return quickly and comfortably back to your normal daily activities. Radiation too can affect the arm and shoulder movement – so the same applies. Start slowly with the mobility exercises, listen to your body, work within a comfortable range and then add in the strength exercises later. Remember to take advice from your doctor who will tell you when you can start exercising again and what is advisable to do.

After my mastectomy and lymph node surgery I was given exercises to start immediately. These were fine as far as they went. A Pilates class is an easy and positive way to regain and maintain movement. You focus on more than the 'problem' area, and not simply protecting it. We all do that with areas we're worried about, however much we try not to. In a matter of weeks I had the full range of movement back. I can move my left arm and shoulder as freely as my right.

Fiona O'Donovan (you can read Fiona's full case study on page 95).

WARM-UP

The warm-up is an important part of your regular routine and should be performed before continuing with any of the exercises at whatever level you are practising. This is because the warming up helps you to become centred, to grow aware of your body alignment and to start the lengthening process that the exercises encourage and require. It also promotes blood flow, joint mobility and enhances concentration. If you find that your joints feel stiff, it's even more important that you do these preliminary moves.

You might like to perform your warm-up in front of a long mirror so that you can keep an eye on your posture. If you're like most of my clients who don't want to look at themselves while they exercise, then you will think this is a dreadful idea, but I can't emphasize enough how useful this can be.

Note: *if you have jumped straight to this warm-up without reading Chapter 5 on postural alignment please read it now so that you know and understand what all the terms used in the following warm-up exercises mean.*

Method

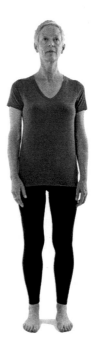

- Stand tall, shoulders stabilized, arms relaxed at your sides.
- Imagine helium balloons are attached to the top of your head and lifting you upwards.
- Lengthen through your spine.
- Fix your gaze on something ahead of you as this will help you to concentrate.
- Perform a few pelvic tilts and find your Neutral Spine (page 32).
- Engage your abdominal muscles/pelvic floor muscles (page 34).
- Breathe in through your nose and into your rib cage (page 39).
- Breathe out through your mouth.
- Repeat the breathing a couple more times and be aware of any muscular tensions in your body — try to consciously relax and let the breathing focus your attention.

NECK

Stiff neck? Try this:

- Perform these warm-up exercises gently and listen to your body. If your neck feels uncomfortable, stop.
- Drop your ear to one shoulder, gently stretching out the other side of your neck and upper back muscles.
- Keep lengthening through your neck.

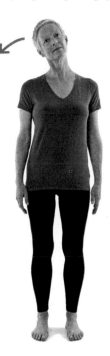 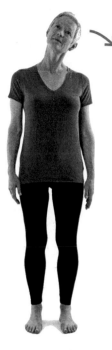 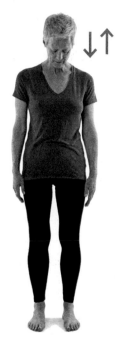

- Lift your head slowly back up to centre – repeat up to 4 times towards that shoulder.

- Perform the exercise to the other shoulder up to 4 times.

- Now drop your chin down on to your chest.
- Gently rotate your neck to one side but don't take it beyond your shoulder.
- Gently rotate to the other side, letting the weight of your head carry it slowly from side to side.
- Repeat two more times either side if you're comfortable to do so, then come back to centre and lift up your head, lengthening through your neck and spine once again.

SHOULDERS

Problems with your shoulders? Take this section gently and slowly, do less rotations if your shoulders feel uncomfortable and don't force anything.

- Rotate your shoulders gently forwards up to 4 times.

- Rotate your shoulders gently backwards up to 4 times.

- Lift your shoulders up around your ears.

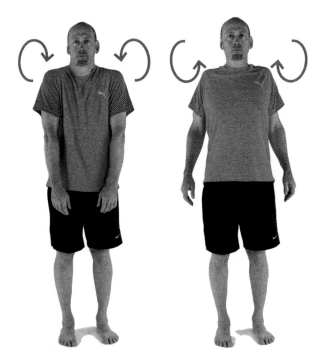
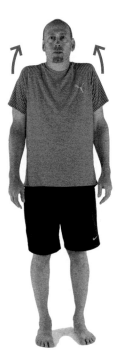

- Take your shoulders back, opening out your chest as you slide your shoulder blades down towards your imaginary back pockets.
- Repeat twice.

SPINAL ROTATION (TWISTING)

Back problems? Only rotate your spine as far as you are comfortable. If you have serious back problems, please take advice from your medical professional about the suitability of rotational exercises.

- Lengthen through your spine.
- Take your right hand and hold your left forearm above your wrist.
- Rotate your left arm to take hold of your right forearm above the wrist.
- Engage your abdominal muscles/pelvic floor muscles.
- Breathe in to prepare.
- Breathe out and rotate your torso to the right, taking your head and neck with you.

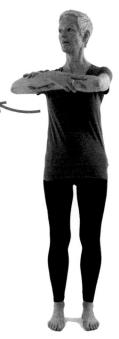

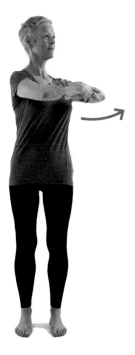

- Concentrate on keeping your pelvis facing forwards as you rotate – it doesn't move with you, it needs to remain stable.
- Keep your shoulders relaxed and down.
- Breathe in and return to centre.
- Breathe out and rotate to the left.

- Breathe in and return to centre.
- Repeat up to 3 times either side.

LATERAL FLEXION (SIDE BENDING)

- Standing tall again in Neutral Spine (page 32), engage your abdominal muscles/pelvic floor muscles.
- Breathe in to prepare.
- Breathe out and slowly slide your hand down the side of your leg, lengthening your fingers as you do so.
- Hold the position.
- Breathe in.
- Imagine you are standing between two panes of glass, so your neck or chin aren't jutting forwards; you will be aligned with your whole body in the same plane.
- Breathe out and return to an upright position, lengthening through your spine as you do so and checking that your abdominal muscles are still engaged.
- Repeat on the other side.

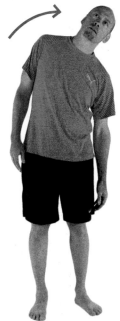 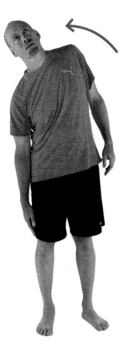

KNEE AND HIP MOBILITY

Is balancing on one leg a challenge?
Try this:

- Take care and keep your toe touching the floor to start with until you feel more confident.

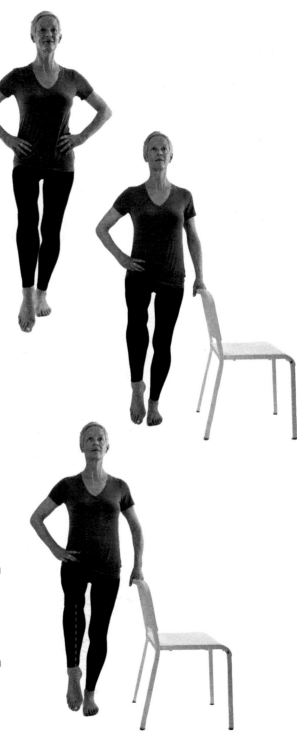

- Standing tall, lengthen through your spine.
- Put both hands on your hips, or one hand on your hip with the other holding on to the back of a chair if you need to, but keeping your shoulders relaxed.
- Engage your abdominal muscles/pelvic floor muscles.
- Breathe naturally for this part of the warm-up because it's more dynamic than the previous movements.
- Lift your knee up in front of you.

- Try not to collapse in your centre, and keep your gaze fixed ahead of you, still lengthening through the spine.
- Take your leg back down to the floor.
- Repeat up to 4 times on both sides.

In this exercise, imagine a vertical line through your knee to your foot, so that it is raised and aligned directly in front of you, not slightly to the side or crossing the centre of your body. If you look at your knee, it should be in line with your second or third toe. Again, if you can stand in front of a mirror for this exercise, it will help you with the placement.

HIP OPENER

- Stand tall, still holding on to the back of the chair if you need it, lengthening through your spine to come into Neutral Spine (page 32), abdominal muscles engaged, arms by your sides, shoulders relaxed.
- Breathe naturally.
- Raise your knee up in front of you.
- Open your hip to the side, taking your leg/knee with you but keeping your pelvis stable. Don't let the pelvis swing back.

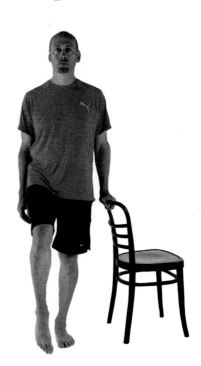

- Bring the leg back to centre and lower to the floor.
- Repeat up to 4 times and then change sides.

ROLL DOWN

Benefits
This is a wonderful, relaxing exercise that can be used as a warm-up. It is also an excellent stretch for your lower back should it be achy or stiff first thing in the morning or after an afternoon of exercise or gardening. It can relieve tired glutes (buttock muscles) or tight hamstrings (back of thighs) after a long walk. The Roll Down improves spinal mobility, encouraging even sequential movement throughout the whole spine, allowing the spinal discs to expand, and developing flexibility of the back and hamstrings. You might like to stick to the basic Roll Down exercise to start with and then add in the progressions for a deeper stretch when you've practised a few times.

BEGINNER
Method
- Stand tall with shoulders relaxed and in Neutral Spine.
- Engage your abdominal muscles/pelvic floor muscles.
- Keep your knees soft and very slightly bent.
- Breathe in to your rib cage to prepare.
- Breathe out as you bring your chin on to your chest.
- Slowly begin to roll yourself down towards the floor. Stop when you come to a comfortable point of tension. If you can't go far, don't worry.

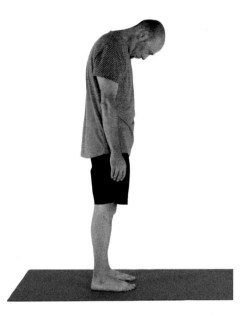

- Let your arms hang loose from your shoulders in front of you.
- Keep your knees slightly bent so that you don't strain your hamstrings if they're feeling a little tight.
- Your neck should be relaxed and your head heavy.
- Imagine you are a rag doll as you gently 'hang', letting everything relax.
- Breathe naturally and hold the 'rag doll' position for a few seconds.
- Breathe into your rib cage.

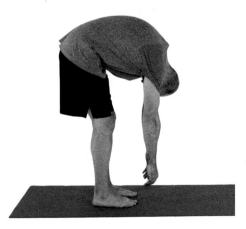

▶▶

- Breathe out and, making sure your abdominal muscles/pelvic floor muscles are engaged to protect your spine, start to uncurl your body vertebrae by vertebrae, slowly building up your spine, strong, straight and tall.
- As you reach the top, keep your chin on your chest until the last second, then uncurl, lengthening through your spine.

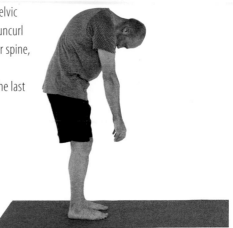

Note:
- Make sure you are bending through your spine and not your hips.
- Keep your weight evenly distributed through both feet: don't lean back into your heels.

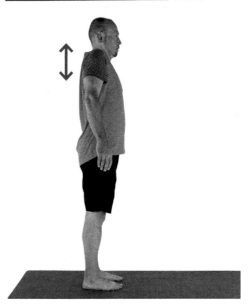

- Breathe naturally and check your posture, lifting your shoulders up around your ears and sending your shoulder blades down into your imaginary back pockets again.
- Check that you're still in Neutral Spine.
- Repeat the Roll Down up to 3 times in total – or as many times as you feel you want to.

Lower back problems? Try this modification:
- If you have any lower back problems at all or you don't feel confident in the 'rag doll' position, you can modify this exercise by placing the palms of your hands on to your thighs. Slide them down your legs as you roll down, supporting your back in the process. If you feel any discomfort at all, stop.

You could also do this exercise resting against a wall:
- Relax your spine against the wall, with your feet a comfortable distance away, hip width apart. Knees slightly bent. Peel your spine off the wall and keep your bottom resting against the wall at the lowest position. Then rebuild your spine against the wall.

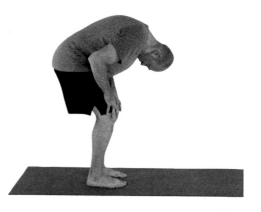

INTERMEDIATE

- For a deeper stretch, when you're in the 'rag doll' position, take the palms of your hands on to your opposite elbows and move your weight gently forwards on to the balls of your feet. But take care you don't overbalance.

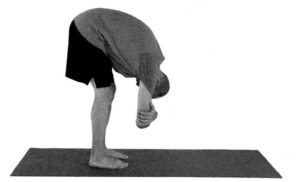

ADVANCED

- Increasing the stretch further, still in the Roll Down, bend one knee gently so that you get a stretch on the other side, and hold that position.
- Straighten your bent knee and then bend the other one, again holding the position for a few seconds.
- Alternate between the two, keeping your feet on the ground, just easing and lengthening the muscles.
- Repeat up to 6 times then come to a standstill.
- Engage your abdominal muscles/pelvic floor muscles.
- Breathe in.
- Breathe out and start to uncurl once again. Take your time and be aware of your alignment.

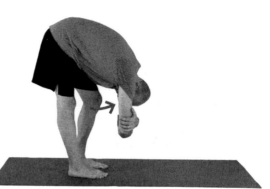

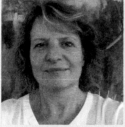

CASE STUDY

Tania Baldwin-Pask
Age: 51
Occupation: Human Rights Advocate
Practised Pilates for: 4 years
Favourite exercise: Roll Down (page 51)

'I started Pilates because I wanted to improve my running and strengthen my pelvic floor muscles. I'm a black belt in Tae Kwon Do, and both that and running require a strong core. I've noticed a huge difference in my core muscles as a result of Pilates. I also have more flexibility – especially because my other sports are contradictory in terms of muscle groups used. And I'm 2cm taller! Pilates is my "me time": deep breathing, slow, deliberate movements – its all very relaxing. It's the best exercise because it offers something to everyone, including people with balance problems.'

Chapter 8

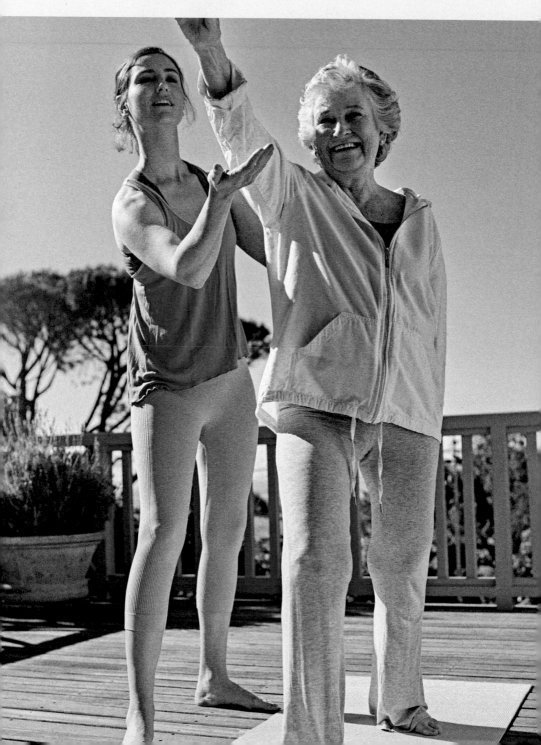

Balance

Benefits of Balance

As we age, our ability to balance declines, so it's very important to practise. To balance well we need to have good **_proprioception_**, coordination, strong ankles and feet (for foot health and strengthening exercises, see Chapter 9). Balance exercises help the brain to recognize and cope with changes in terrain when we walk. The exercises will also help with concentration. You might find that as you practise these exercises you discover that your balance is better on one side of your body than the other as we all have a dominant side.

Try to incorporate some kind of balance exercise into your everyday life – maybe stand on one leg while you're waiting for the kettle to boil, brushing your teeth or waiting in the bus queue. But if you're not confident about your ability to balance, please do be careful and make sure there is something that you can hang on to.

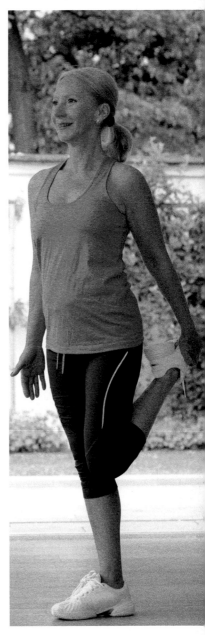

RESEARCH

In a research study called 'Integrating Pilates Exercise into an Exercise Program for 65+ Year-Old Women To Reduce Falls' at the School of Physical Education and Sports at Mugla University, Turkey, it was concluded that Pilates-based exercises were shown to improve dynamic balance, reaction time and muscle strength in the elderly.

BALANCE PRACTICE

Method

- Stand tall, lengthening through your spine, in Neutral Spine.
- Engage your abdominal muscles/pelvic floor muscles.
- Fix your gaze and concentrate on something ahead of you to help you balance.
- Slowly lift one knee directly in front of you a little way.
- Hold your balance, standing on one leg in this position and count to 5 to start with. If you can only manage a few seconds, don't worry, keep trying and it will improve. You can increase the amount of time you hold your balance as and when you feel more confident – aim to count up to 20 slowly.
- Try not to hold your breath and breathe naturally. Keep your waist long and even on both sides of the body.
- Lower the leg and change sides, repeating the balance for another count of 5.

Wobbling too much? Too challenging? Try this:

- During the exercises, if you find that you wobble a lot, hold on to something with a very light touch, and lift your hand from time to time.

- Or: touch the floor with your toe before taking your foot away and balancing. Each time you wobble, return your toe back to the floor for a second.

Take it slowly, and if you're holding on to something, every now and again let go; you'll find that your body will soon get the message and your balance will improve. If you do these exercises in front of a mirror, you can make sure that your pelvis stays level and doesn't tilt to one side as you lift your leg, which could be a sign of gluteal weakness (see page 146 for the Shoulder Bridge exercise which will highlight this problem if you have it and also help to improve it).

Balance exercises are also good for all lower limb injuries.

Good balance? Try this:
If you're confident with the first balance exercise, you can progress on to this more challenging version.

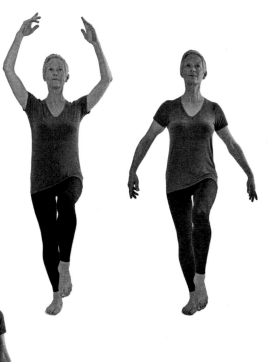

- Return to the first side, raise your leg and find your balance, engage your abdominals and lengthen through your spine again.
- Breathe in and lift both arms up and above your head.
- Breathe out and lower them to the sides of your body.
- Repeat the arm sequence once more, still standing on one leg.
- Change sides and repeat.

And if the above is easy, you might like to try the exercise with your eyes closed. Just please make sure that you don't fall!
- Keep the leg low to start with and touch the floor with your toe to get started.

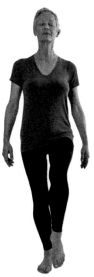

- Hold for a few seconds and then increase the amount of time you keep your eyes closed. This can be very challenging and demonstrates how important our visual sense is to maintaining balance.

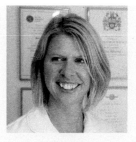

PROFESSIONAL ADVICE

Osteopath Jane Kaushal says:

'Many injuries to the ankle and knees arise because of poor balance. If you have ever sprained your ankle, the proprioceptors (joint position sensors) in your ankle ligaments will not be as efficient at detecting where your ankle is in space. This means that other parts of your lower leg take the strain instead, especially when you are walking on uneven ground. Pilates can improve proprioception, which will reduce unnecessary strain on joints and help prevent injury. Your ability to balance decreases naturally with age so you need to work to maintain or even improve this. Importantly, improved proprioception and balance will help to prevent falls, and Pilates can certainly help in that respect. Falling in later life is bad news for many reasons, so anything we can do to prevent this is very helpful indeed!'

Chapter 9

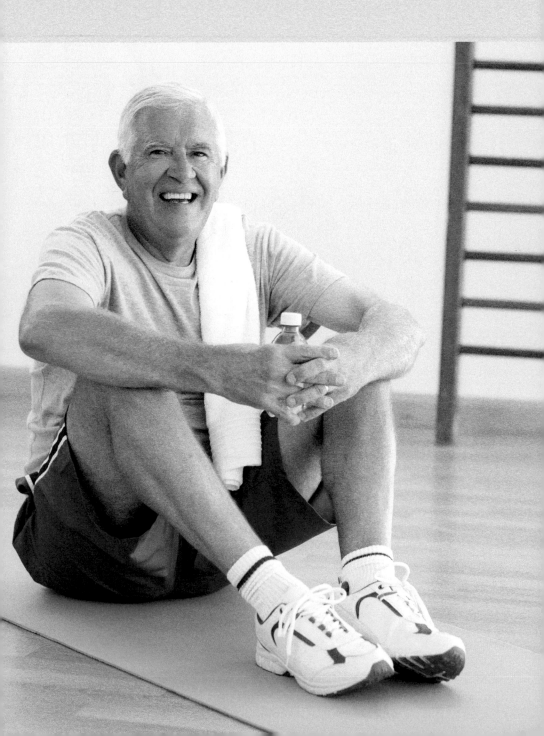

Foot health and strengthening exercises

When planning a regular exercise routine, foot strengthening and stretching exercises are probably not one of the first things you think to include. But they are vital for us as we age, our joints stiffen and muscle mass decreases. At the risk of stating the obvious, our feet receive a huge amount of impact when we walk about, jog or play sport, and they also play an essential part in stabilization. I include these exercises in all of my Pilates classes. Not only will they strengthen your feet, but also the muscles, ligaments and tendons attached.

Plantar fasciitis can be a common and painful complaint as we age, causing heel pain that makes walking uncomfortable. We lose some of the strength and springiness in the sole of the foot as the tendons lose their stretch, which in turn makes it harder for the foot to absorb impact, making us more prone to this condition. But by practising the foot exercises regularly and keeping our feet healthy, plantar fasciitis can be prevented. I also include an Ankle Mobility and Foot Stretch exercise in this chapter. All of these exercises can be practised whenever you get the opportunity, preferably in bare feet.

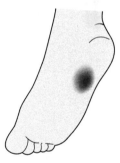

Plantar fasciitis causes heel pain and makes walking uncomfortable.

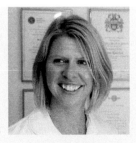

PROFESSIONAL ADVICE

Osteopath Jane Kaushal says:

"'Use it or lose it' is even more relevant when it comes to foot flexibility and health in later life. After the age of 60 many people's feet become stiff or even rigid if they do nothing to maintain foot health. Rigid feet do not balance properly as they can't adapt to the surface they are on, and the intrinsic muscles within the feet become very weak. Feet are therefore at the mercy of external forces and can make bunion deformities or plantar fascia pain more likely to develop. Any balancing and stretching exercise in bare feet is helpful, and Pilates is ideal. It will move the feet and ankles through a full range of movement and maintain the strength of the small muscles deep in the feet. In addition, I would recommend standing on one foot when you brush your teeth – left foot in the morning and the right foot before you go to bed!'

ACHILLES AND CALF MUSCLE STRENGTHENER

Benefits

The *Achilles tendon* stretches from the bone of your heel at the back of your leg to your calf muscles that sit just above it. These calf muscles can become quite tight and stiff and so stretching and strengthening them is vital to keep them healthy and prevent injury.

Balance not good? Try this:

- Hold on to a chair when you perform these exercises if you're worried about toppling. And see Chapter 8 for more balance practice.

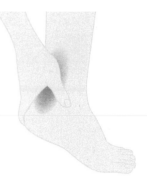

The Achilles – this tendon connects the calf muscles to the heel bone.

Method

- Stand tall, lengthening through your spine.
- Slowly begin to pedal up and down on the balls of your feet – come right up, nearly on to your toes if you can.
- Repeat up to 10 times in total, as long as it is comfortable to do so.

- Now come up on to the balls of both feet together and balance. Hold the position up to the count of 4. If this is challenging, then just hold for as long as you can and increase the time once you feel confident.

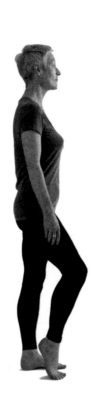

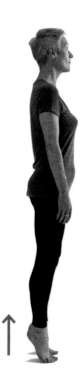

- Lower both heels back down to the mat as slowly as you can.
- Repeat up to 4 times, keeping the movement slow and controlled.

- Perform 5 fast heel lifts – feel those calf muscles working! You can increase the repetitions to 10 if you're comfortable to do so.

BRAIN GYM FOR FEET

Benefits

This simple exercise will not only stretch and strengthen your feet but also challenge your stability, coordination and concentration.

Method

- Stand tall, lengthening through the spine.
- Rise up on to the ball of your right foot only.

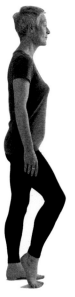

- Now come up on to the ball of your left foot.

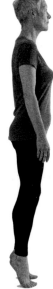

- Take your right heel slowly down to the floor.

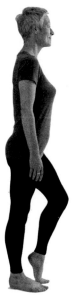

- Take your left heel down.

- Repeat the moves up to 5 times in total and then change sides, starting on the left.

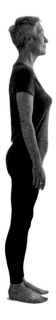

HEELS AND TOES

Benefits

The following exercises strengthen the feet and lower legs, improve mobility of the toes and the inner foot muscles, stretch the arches and improve overall coordination.

Method

- Stand tall, lengthening through the spine.
- Walk forwards on your toes for up to 10 steps.
- Walk backwards on your toes for up to 10 steps.

- Now walk forwards on your heels for up to 10 steps.
- Walk backwards on your heels for up to 10 steps.

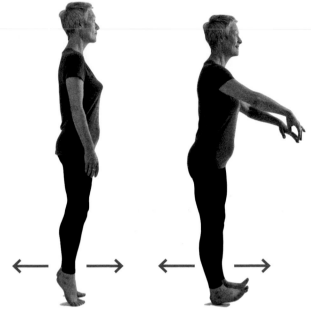

- Repeat the sequence several times.
- Come to a standstill and, lengthening through your spine, lift your toes up off the floor.

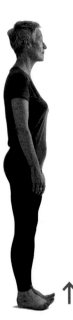

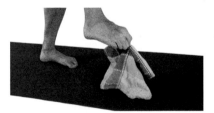

- Hold for a few seconds and then fold your toes in the opposite direction – if you want to make this a more challenging exercise, see if you can pick up a small towel, a pen or marbles with your folded toes!
- Repeat a few times if you're comfortable to do so but be aware of what else your body is doing – make sure your fists aren't clenching at the same time.
- Of course, these last two exercises can be performed while sitting down if preferred.

ANKLE MOBILITY

Benefits

This is a simple but important exercise to achieve and maintain full range of movement and improve strength in the ankles and feet. As already mentioned, your feet and ankles have to withstand the impact of walking or standing, and this exercise will help them to do so. You can also perform this exercise standing up if you prefer, as part of the balance routine (page 56) or follow on from the previous foot exercises – but don't forget to hang on to something if your balance isn't too good. The pointing and flexing of the foot improves flexibility and also stretches and lengthens the muscles of the front and back of the leg. If you're short of time, instead of lying on your back, perform the exercises while you're sitting at your desk and don't forget to include the previous two exercises of scrunching and lifting your toes as well.

Method

- Lie on your back.
- Place a block or small cushion under your head to keep your neck and spine aligned.
- Bend your knees.
- Place your feet in line with your hips.
- Perform a few pelvic tilts and come into Neutral Spine.
- Engage your abdominal muscles/pelvic floor muscles.
- Breathe naturally and raise one leg up into Table Top.

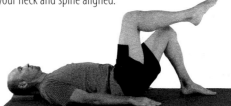

- Place your hands lightly around your raised thigh to support the leg.
- Rotate your ankle very slowly in one direction 6 times, and then reverse it.

- Return your foot to centre, then alternate pointing your toes and flexing your foot 6 times.
- Change legs and repeat the exercise on the other side.

Note:
- Try to draw a full circle with your toes when rotating from your ankle.
- Keep the knee and lower leg stable. Don't let it circle with your foot.
- Relax your shoulders. Be aware of the rest of your body – is it trying to join in?

FOOT MASSAGE

Benefits

If you've been standing all day or been for a long walk, shopping expedition or other activity, your feet can become very tired, achy and sore. Using a massage ball, foot roller or even a tennis ball to massage the underneath of your foot can improve the circulation, reduce discomfort and be very relaxing. And of course you can perform these standing up, lying down or sitting on the sofa watching TV, along with the other foot exercises in this chapter. Massaging your feet this way can also help to relieve and reduce symptoms of plantar fasciitis.

Method:

- Place the ball under the sole of your foot.
- Roll from toe to heel for a minute or so.
- Rotate the massage ball first one way and then reverse and go the other way.

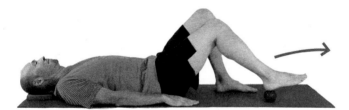

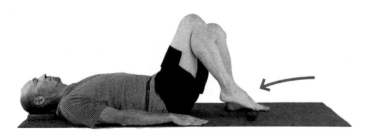

- Repeat several times – if you find an especially sore spot, spend more time on it.
- Don't forget to do the other foot!

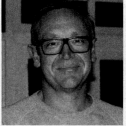

CASE STUDY

Warren Jacobs
Age: 45
Occupation: Designer
Practised Pilates for: 1 year
Favourite exercise: Heel and foot stretches

'My employer fortunately arranged classes in the office and I was acutely aware that I needed to stretch because I run and kept straining my heels and calves. However, this has eased since I've started attending the Pilates class. At the end of the session and for a day or two afterwards my posture feels much better. I don't feel so hunched. I have a lot more energy and Pilates is allowing me to run better – both of these things together are making significant improvements to how I feel. Like me, many of my friends are tied to their computer all day, Pilates is a fantastic remedy for the hunched posture this causes us to adopt. It's given me a way to counterbalance the effects that my job has on my flexibility and posture.'

Chapter 10

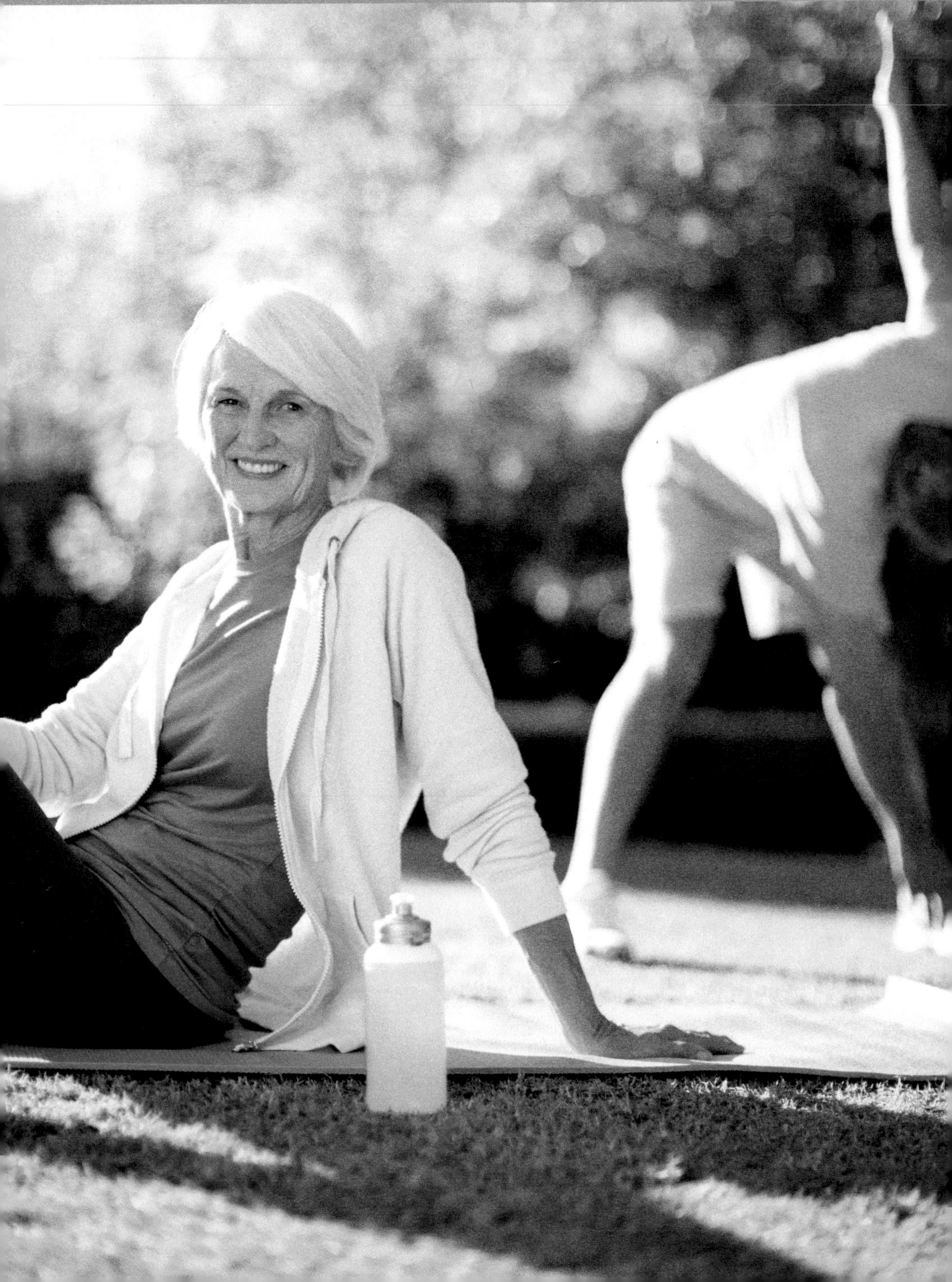

Mat Pilates exercises

In this next section of the book you will find all the main mat Pilates exercises. Some of the following exercises are suitable for all levels of experience and fitness and are labelled as such, while others offer a Beginner, Intermediate and Advanced version. If you've come to this book terrified of exercise, not sure what would be the best place to start or you've been injured, are recovering from an operation or are feeling frail, begin with the Starter Pack exercises on page 68 before you do anything else. Practise these and they will give you confidence to move on to the Beginner exercises.

Following the Starter Pack you will find some simple stretches. You may recognize these as being similar to yoga poses. These are particularly good when performed after completion of one of the main exercises as a relief stretch. It's worth familiarizing yourself with them so that you don't have to keep finding the page where the instructions are.

For those of you who have practised some Pilates before and are already fairly active, then have a go at the Intermediate exercises. I'll leave it up to you to decide when you feel ready to try the more challenging advanced ones – suffice to say, make sure you can perform the Intermediate exercises without compromising your alignment or precision before you move on to the Advanced. At the back of the book you'll find some suggested Pilates routines which will help you mix and match the exercises, then once you are familiar with them you can begin to choose your own routines to suit your personal needs.

It's important to note that just because an exercise looks or feels easy, it doesn't mean that it isn't worth doing. All the exercises, at whatever level, are in this book because they will help improve your strength, flexibility, coordination, balance and posture, and keep you going on! Too often we jump to the more challenging exercises in the hope that they will accelerate improvements – it doesn't work like that. The 'easier' exercises build a strong foundation for you to grow your practice from. They will continually encourage you to revisit the Pilates principles (page 21) as you learn the fundamentals and hone your technique. That way you'll get the most out of every level. Don't start with the Advanced exercises if you haven't performed and understood the exercises for beginners.

Before some of the exercises I have also noted certain cautions that may need to be considered. These apply to any specific problems you may have, and where it might be advisable to either adapt the exercise or omit it altogether. Again, if in doubt, please take advice from a medical practitioner or specialist in relation to your own specific problem.

But whatever you do, as you work through the exercises, enjoy the feeling of becoming stronger, more flexible, coordinated and youthful.

STARTER PACK

This section is for those of you who have done very little exercise, are feeling nervous about starting Pilates or are recovering from surgery or illness. Have a go at the following sequence of exercises (always make sure you've completed the warm-up beforehand) and when you've mastered these you can have a go at the rest of the exercises in the book. But do start with the ones designed for beginners and progress slowly, taking care to listen to your body as you perform them.

> Have you warmed up? Return to Chapter 7 for the gentle warm-up exercises.

LEG SLIDE

Benefits

This simple exercise is a great way of training your torso (particularly your pelvis and spine) to stay stable while you move your legs. It's also a good exercise for hip mobility and will improve your coordination.

Method

- Lie down on your back.
- Place a block or small cushion under your head to keep your neck and spine aligned.
- Take your arms down by your sides and keep them relaxed.

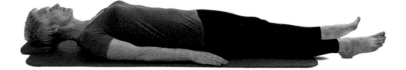

- Bend your knees.
- Place your feet in line with your hips.
- Make sure you're in Neutral Spine – perform a few pelvic tilts to find the correct position and then relax.

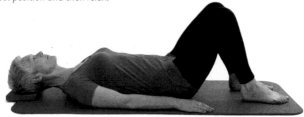

- Engage your abdominal muscles/pelvic floor muscles.
- Breathe in to your ribcage to prepare.
- Breathe out through your mouth and gently slide one leg away from you, extending it along the mat.

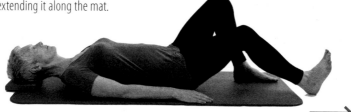

- Breathe in and return your leg, sliding it back to the start position.
- Repeat with the other leg.
- Continue for up to 8 repetitions.

Note:
- Be aware of any pelvic movement – is your pelvis tilting as you move the leg? Try to keep it stable and in Neutral Spine.
- Keep your abdominal muscles engaged and the rest of your body heavy and relaxed, with your shoulders softly down in your imaginary back pockets.
- Concentrate on your breathing to help the exercise flow.

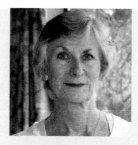

CASE STUDY

Julia Hick
Age: 62
Practised Pilates for: 7 years
Favourite exercise: Scissors (page 158)

'I play tennis on a regular basis and now find I have more stamina and move faster on court. There's also less pain in my hip. Many of the exercises were recommended to me by my physiotherapist. I now make more effort to try to "stand tall" as well. I've been told by lots of people I look more toned and have a younger figure than 10 years ago, and I'm pleased to admit I feel happiest in my life now – feeling fit and healthy with a good positive outlook in general. I like the classes because I'm with like-minded people in a non-judgemental group as there's no competition to be better than others. I always finish the session feeling relaxed and fitter.'

NECK CURL-UP

Benefits

These gentle Curl-Ups will introduce you to activating the abdominal muscles while you raise your head, neck and shoulders. You will need to be able to do this in many of the exercises. Neck Curl-Ups target the rectus abdominis, the potential six-pack muscles, as well as working the neck flexors. However, if you have osteoporosis or osteopenia in your neck, please take advice as to whether the flexion movement is safe. Flexion is lifting your head and bringing your chin towards your chest. If in doubt, leave it out, and check with a medical practitioner before commencing.

Method

- Lie down on your back.
- Bend your knees with your feet in line with your hips.
- Place a block or small cushion under your head to keep your neck and spine aligned.
- Place one hand on your abdomen and put the other lightly under your head.

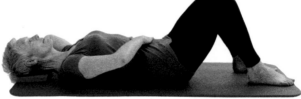

- Make sure you are in Neutral Spine.
- Engage your abdominal muscles/pelvic floor muscles.
- Breathe in to prepare.
- Breathe out and gently raise your head, supported by your hand, lengthening and flexing your neck, looking down towards your thighs.

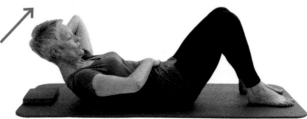

- Breathe in and hold the position.
- Breathe out and lower yourself back down to the starting position.
- Repeat up to 3 times and change hands and then continue for another 3 repetitions.

Note:

- By placing your hand on your tummy you will be able to feel the muscles working underneath your palm as you curl up.
- If you feel your abdominal muscles start to bulge, return back down to the floor. Imagine 'scooping your abdominals' and maintaining a long torso.

- Always keep the abdominal muscles activated – pull them in before you move so that you are centred and stable and your abdominal muscles won't dome.

- When you've completed the repetitions, come into a Full Body Stretch.

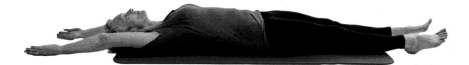

CASE STUDY

Ann Gordon Cummings
Age: 69
Occupation: Dog walker
Practised Pilates for: 3.5 years
Favourite exercise: Side Kick (page 110)

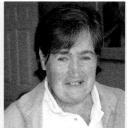

'Since taking up Pilates my elbow is so much stronger, after it grew 'stalactites' in the joint. Pilates has really helped, particularly the push-ups – I could only do 3 or 4 when I started and now I can do 12. I have also suffered from a thigh injury and since taking up Pilates I no longer have any pain. Side-lying Pilates exercises help no end.

I used to sit at a desk for a long time each day but now I am a dog walker and I walk at least 3 miles a day. I now remember to stand tall when walking and not lean forward. I'm always much looser after Pilates and I particularly notice it when I walk the dogs after class. I feel a lot better for practising Pilates.'

HIP ROLL

Benefits

A great exercise to perform after a long day sitting, or an active day of walking, cycling, gardening or other activity. It will relieve tension in a tight lower back and helps realign the spine while challenging the abdominal muscles and the *obliques* (waist muscles).

Method

- Lie on your back with your knees bent, legs and feet together.
- Take your arms out to the sides, relaxed and placed just below shoulder level with palms facing up.

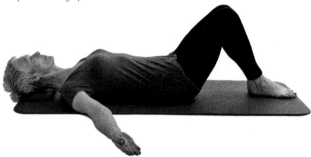

- Engage your abdominal muscles/pelvic floor muscles.
- Breathe in to prepare.
- Breathe out and drop both your knees together towards the floor on one side.

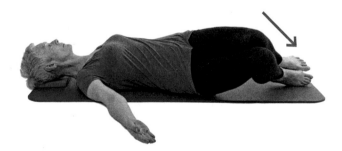

- Breathe in and hold the position.
- Breathe out as you lift them back up to centre.
- Repeat to the other side.
- Repeat up to 4 times each side.

Note:
- Try to keep the opposite shoulder on the mat.
- Keep your knees and legs connected throughout the exercise.
- Make sure you're using your abdominal muscles and not your back muscles when you lift your knees up off the floor – you will feel the difference.

ONE LEG KNEE FOLD STARTER

Have you warmed up?
Return to Chapter 7
for the gentle warm-up
exercises.

Benefits

This exercise will acquaint you with the Table Top position used in many of these exercises. It will also gently challenge your core muscles, teaching you to keep your pelvis and spine stable while moving your leg.

Method

- Lie on your back with your knees bent.
- Place a small cushion or block under your head to keep your neck and spine aligned.
- Place your feet in line with your hips.
- Take your arms down by your sides and keep them relaxed.

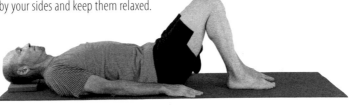

- Perform a few pelvic tilts and come into Neutral Spine.
- Engage your abdominal muscles/pelvic floor muscles.
- Breathe in to prepare.
- Breathe out and float one of your legs up into Table Top – so your shin is parallel to the ceiling and your knee sits above your hip. Point your toes if it's comfortable to do so.

- Hold that position for a few breaths making sure your abdominal muscles are engaged. Check that the rest of your body is relaxed – shoulders are heavy and released into the mat.
- Breathe in to your ribcage.
- Breathe out and lower the leg, with control, slowly back down to the floor.
- Repeat on the other side and complete 6 repetitions in total, alternating legs.

Note:

- When you raise your leg, check for any movement in the pelvic area. Try and keep the pelvis and spine stable and in neutral.
- When you return the leg back down to the floor, pay particular attention to any arching that might occur in your lower back. Engage those abdominal muscles and keep in Neutral Spine.

KNEE DROP STARTER

Benefits
This is a great exercise for hip mobility and encourages pelvic stability, challenging the core muscles. So be aware when you're performing the exercise of any movement and try to correct it.

Method
- Lie on your back.
- Place a block or small cushion under your head to keep your neck and spine aligned.
- Take your arms down by your sides and keep them relaxed.
- Bend your knees.
- Place your feet in line with your hips.

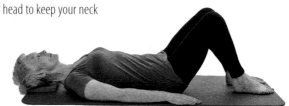

- Perform a few gentle pelvic tilts and come into Neutral Spine.
- Engage your abdominal muscles/pelvic floor muscles.
- Breathe in to prepare.
- Breathe out and gently drop one knee slowly out to the side – your foot will roll onto its outer edge.

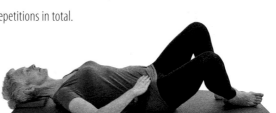

- Breathe in and return your knee to centre.
- Alternate the legs and complete up to 10 repetitions in total.

Is your pelvis rocking? Try this:
- Place your hands over your hips so that you can be aware of any movement and correct it.

Not challenging enough? Try the progression for this exercise on page 179.

Note:
- Only take your knee as far as it will comfortably go.
- Be aware of any rocking movement that might be going on with the pelvis. Try to avoid the weight of the leg pulling the pelvis to that side. Stay level and neutral.
- Keep your abdominal muscles engaged and your opposite knee stable.
- Use your breathing to help with concentration.
- Be aware of any tensions in the rest of the body.

SINGLE LEG SIDE KICK

Benefits

The Single Leg Side Kick will work your core muscles, specifically your oblique (waist) muscles and hip area. The stronger the oblique muscles, the less likelihood of pelvis and hip problems.

Method

- Lie on your side.
- Lengthen your underneath arm directly under your head and place your head on your block or small cushion which you can balance between the upper part of your arm and head. This will keep your neck and spine aligned.

Note: *If you have had a recent hip replacement or have osteoporosis, take care with this exercise and please make sure that you don't let your top leg cross over your bottom leg to the floor. You could place a cushion underneath the top leg to keep it at hip height. If unsure of the suitability of this exercise, please omit or check with your health professional.*

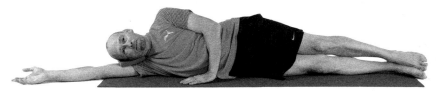

- Lengthen both legs along the mat, one on top of the other in a straight line.
- Glance down towards your feet, check that your hips, knees and ankles are aligned on top of each other.
- Place your other hand in front of your torso on the floor for support.
- Engage your abdominal muscles/pelvic floor muscles.
- Breathe in to prepare.
- As you breathe out, raise your top leg in a straight line, with your foot flexed, facing forwards. Think about length rather than height. Only go as high as you can keep the waist long.

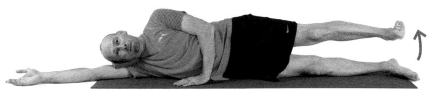

- Breathe in and hold the raised position.
- As you breathe out, slowly lower the leg, with control back down to join the underneath leg.
- Repeat up to 10 times.
- Turn over, and perform the exercise on the other side.

SWAN DIVE ON FOREARMS

Benefits

The Swan Dive exercise strengthens the mid/upper back and abdominal muscles. This introduction to the main exercise will help open out the chest area and strengthen the middle of your back (see thoracic spine, page 30), so that as you age your posture remains upright and strong.

Method

- Lie down on your front.
- Place a block or small cushion under your forehead – this is to keep your neck and spine aligned.
- Bend your arms so that your elbows are level with your shoulders and resting on the floor.
- Place your legs hip-distance apart with your toes slightly turned in.

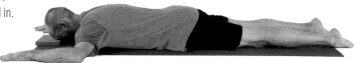

- Engage your abdominal muscles/pelvic floor muscles.
- Breathe in to your ribcage to prepare.
- Breathe out as you gently raise your chest up with forearms still on the floor. Keep your neck lengthened in line with your spine. You don't have to come up too far – just a little way.
- Keep the arms light. Try not to push down hard on the floor, you want your back muscles to work.

- Breathe in at the top.
- Breathe out as you lower yourself slowly back to the floor.
- Repeat up to 6 times in total as long as you are comfortable to do so.

When you've completed this exercise, come into Cat Stretch so that you stretch your back in the opposite way to the way you've been working. There is more information about this stretch and other useful relief stretches in the next section.

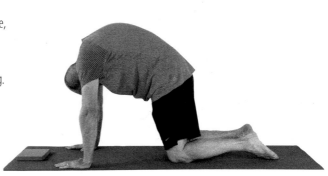

STRETCHY PILATES EXERCISES

Now you have completed the Starter Pack, and as long as you feel comfortable with it, move on to familiarising yourself with the following stretches (you will have performed a couple of them already) before attempting the beginners' exercises. If in doubt of suitability, come back to the Starter Pack until you feel comfortable and confident to continue.

It's worth familiarizing yourself with this section of the book as these are often used as relief stretches after many of the mat Pilates exercises. They also stand alone and are great for improving flexibility and providing relaxation for tired muscles.

CAT STRETCH

Benefits

This is a wonderful yoga-based stretch which you may already be familiar with. It is also an excellent spinal mobilizer, especially if you have a tight lower back. As already mentioned in the introduction to this section of the book you'll see that I've suggested performing this exercise as a relief stretch at the end of some of the exercises, especially in the Back Series: it's a good way of stretching the spine in the opposite direction to the way in which you've been working. The Cat Stretch also works the abdominal muscles.

Note: when you're kneeling, if your knees are a little uncomfortable, put a cushion under each one to take some pressure off. The same applies to wrists.

Method
- Come on to all fours.
- Align your hands under your shoulders and your knees under your hips.

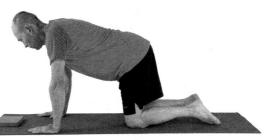

- Engage your abdominal muscles/pelvic floor muscles.
- Breathe in to prepare.
- Breathe out as you slowly and gently arch your back up towards the ceiling, dropping your head and neck – like a cat hissing!

Note:
- You can hold the stretch for as long as you feel you need to.
- Breathe naturally and feel the muscles lengthening in your back as you do so.

- Hold the stretch as you breathe in again.
- Breathe out and return your spine back to neutral.
- Repeat 3 times or more.

EXTENDED CHILD'S POSE

Benefits

This is another yoga-based stretch suitable for aching shoulders and lower back, which can be performed as a relaxation stretch between exercises. It's also a wonderful position to rest in as it lengthens the spine and releases tension.

Method

- Come on to all fours with your knees under your hips and hands aligned under your shoulders.
- Sit back and let your buttocks rest on your heels.
- Lengthen your arms out in front of you, palms pressing down, and let your head rest on the floor.
- Hold the position.

- Breathe in through your nose and in to your ribcage and then slowly out through your mouth. Stay focused as you repeat for up to 5 breaths, as long as you are comfortable in this position, relaxing into it — remember you can always modify (see suggestions towards the end of this exercise). Stretch your arms as far forwards as you can to lengthen the muscles and stretch the upper back.

Note:
- You might find that your back won't let go if it's very tight as it will be protecting itself — so take time with this exercise and don't force anything. If in any doubt, modify.

Tight back? Stiff knees? Try these:
- A tight lower back can prevent you from comfortably sitting back on your heels, so try placing a cushion on your calves and gently sink your bottom down on to it.

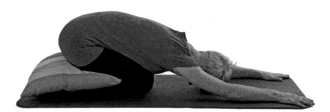

- Stiff knees can also make this position uncomfortable, so try placing a rolled-up towel in the crook of your knee to relieve the tension as you sit gently back.

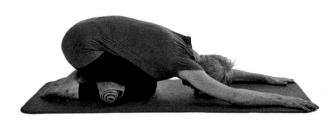

- If you find it challenging to get into the full position, move your knees apart a little but try to keep your toes touching. This will enable you to sink down lower and in between your legs, to rest on the floor – in this position your **adductors** (inner thighs) will also get a stretch.

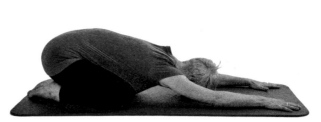

Note: *if your knees or your lower back are extremely tight, please take care or take a look at the modified version on page 78. But if you have serious knee problems, avoid this exercise and instead lie on your side curled forwards.*

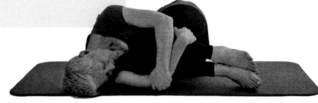

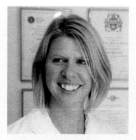

PROFESSIONAL ADVICE

Osteopath Jane Kaushal says:

'We all know that there are many benefits of exercise as we get older. We know that we must keep our heart and lungs working and avoid unnecessary weight gain, but people often forget that strength, balance and flexibility are also of primary importance. Going for a walk or a swim is a wonderful thing to do for lots of reasons, and please do continue doing this and more, but these activities will not necessarily help a great deal with strength, balance and flexibility. That is where Pilates comes in. If you want to look after all aspects of musculoskeletal health, regular Pilates, combined with other physical activity that you enjoy, is the answer.'

COBRA STRETCH

Benefits

This is a yoga-inspired exercise to stretch and open out the chest, abdominal muscles and the hips. During a Pilates session we are often working our abdominal muscles hard. They need to stretch but it's not a part of the anatomy that we often think of stretching. This exercise also strengthens and mobilizes the spine. You should feel this in your upper and mid back, and not in your lower back at all. If you feel any sensation in your lower back, keep it low down. Imagine lengthening the lower back not compressing it.

Method

- Lie on your front.
- Take your arms out to the side and bend your elbows up to the same height as your shoulders.
- Place the palms down.

- Engage your abdominal muscles/pelvic floor muscles.
- Breathe in to prepare.
- Breathe out and gently lift your chest slowly off the floor and extend the elbows, placing your weight on your hands.
- Lift all the way up to your pelvis, if you can, keeping length in your neck and spine and fixing your gaze ahead.

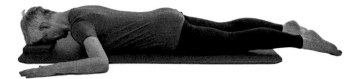

- Breathe in as you hold the stretch.
- Breathe out and slowly lower yourself back down to the floor.
- Repeat up to 6 times, holding for longer at the top if it feels comfortable to do so.

Tough on your back? Try this:
- Bend your elbows if you feel the stretch is too strong for your back.

Note:
- Keep your abdominal muscles engaged and your hips on the floor.
- Relax your shoulders and lengthen your neck, keeping it aligned.
- Concentrate on your breathing to help the movements flow.

FULL BODY STRETCH

And finally, this lengthening stretch often comes at the end of an exercise. It needs no instruction other than to lie on your back and lengthen through the spine. Enjoy the feeling of lengthening the body from the tip of your fingertips to the tip of your toes!

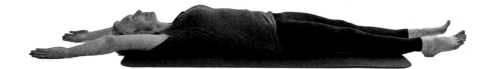

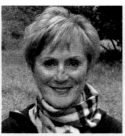

CASE STUDY

Sarah Deriaz
Age: 65
Occupation: Director of a commercial property agency
Practised Pilates for: 3 years
Favourite exercises: exercises that stretch my back

'I play golf twice a week and my upper body rotation and balance has improved since practising Pilates. Some of the stretches we use in Pilates are a great help for warming up before a golf match. I'm also more aware of standing and sitting tall now and often think of engaging my core muscles. I'd recommend Pilates to anyone looking for a full body workout without the aerobic intensity of other exercise. After doing gym work, steps, spinning, etc., Pilates is refreshingly calm, more about strengthening, stretching and concentrating on small movements, so much more intense and effective. I also enjoy the social stimulus and challenge of staying strong. It's given me confidence that I will age well if I continue to practise.'

THE MAIN MAT PILATES EXERCISES

Choose the level that best suits your ability. If you're not sure where to begin, turn to Chapter 12 for a list of suggested routines. Take your time to work through them and familiarize yourself with the different levels and what best suits your ability.

SWIMMING

Benefits

The Swimming exercise encourages torso and spinal stability while moving the arms and legs. We need this stability as we move about our everyday lives. Your core muscles have to constantly stabilize your pelvis when moving around, walking or performing a sporting activity. This exercise teaches the core muscles to work together and provide enough strength for us to stay upright and stable. It also, like most Pilates exercises, lengthens the back, arm and leg muscles, especially the hip flexors (these bend the hip when walking, jogging or climbing a hill, for example) and hamstrings (back of the thighs) that are notorious for becoming tight especially if you sit down a lot. Start with the beginners' version and if that feels comfortable, progress to the intermediate before having a go at the advanced exercise.

BEGINNER

Method

• Lie on your front with your hands one on top of the other supporting your forehead.

Note: *before attempting any of the exercises it is important that you follow the warm-up and include the Roll Down (pages 44–53).*

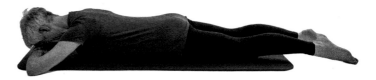

• Engage your abdominal muscles/pelvic floor muscles, feeling the abdominal muscles lifting up off the floor. Try to keep them there.
• Breathe in through your nose to prepare.
• Breathe out through your mouth and raise one leg just a little way off the ground. Lengthen it, pointing your toes.

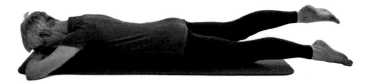

- Breathe in and hold the lengthened position.
- Breathe out and lower the leg to the ground.
- Repeat up to 4 times each side.
- Come into Cat Stretch (page 77) followed by Extended Child's Pose (page 78).

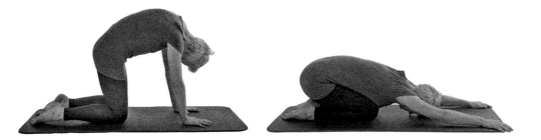

INTERMEDIATE

- Lie on your front. Place your forehead on a block or small cushion with your arms lengthened in front as if you're about to dive into a swimming pool.

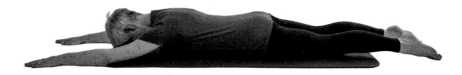

- Engage your abdominal muscles/pelvic floor muscles, feeling the abdominal muscles lifting up off the floor. Try to keep them there.
- Breathe in to prepare.
- Breathe out, raise and lengthen your right arm and left leg, keeping them parallel to the floor, lengthening from fingers to toes.
- Lift your head just a little, keeping your neck and spine aligned.

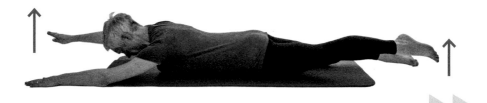

- Breathe in as you hold the position.
- Breathe out as you lower your limbs, head and neck back down to the ground.
- Repeat on the other side and then keep going until you've completed up to 6 repetitions in total – 3 each side.

- Come into Cat Stretch (page 77) followed by Extended Child's Pose (page 78).

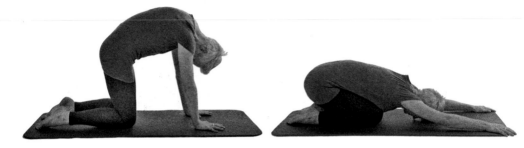

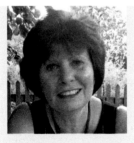

CASE STUDY

Joanna Tinker
Age: 57
Practised Pilates for: 10 years
Favourite exercise: Cat Stretch because it really eases back pain (page 77)

'I started Pilates because I had bad back pain and needed to strengthen my core muscles and pelvic floor. I also have mild arthritis in my back and hips. Since practising Pilates my posture has improved, my back is stronger and I get less backache. I have better flexibility and less pain in my joints, so fewer anti-inflammatory tablets required. I use the breathing when the going gets tough – so it lowers stress levels too!'

SWIMMING INTO BACK EXTENSION

ADVANCED

Please make sure you have warmed up the spine beforehand – perform the Roll Down exercise (page 51)

Method

- Lie on your front, place your forehead on a block or small cushion with your arms lengthened above your head as if you're about to dive into a swimming pool.

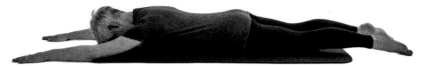

- Engage your abdominal muscles/pelvic floor muscles, feeling your abdominal muscles lifting up off the floor.
- Breathe in to prepare.
- Breathe out, raise and lengthen both your arms and legs, keeping them parallel to the floor.
- Lift your head, keeping your neck and spine aligned.
- Hold for up to 5 seconds if you are comfortable to do so, but remember to breathe naturally in this position.
- Breathe in to your ribcage again.

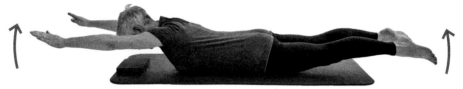

- Breathe out as you lower yourself back to the ground.
- Repeat up to 4 times in total and then come into Cat Stretch (page 77) followed by Extended Child's Pose (page 78).

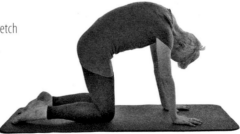

Note:

- Keep your abdominal muscles lifted and engaged.
- Make sure you don't overextend your back: you shouldn't feel any compression in the lumbar spine at all.
- Concentrate and keep focused on your breathing and alignment.

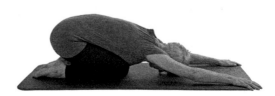

SWAN DIVE

Benefits

Swan Dive strengthens the mid/upper back and abdominal muscles. Those rounded, forward-slumped shoulders that can get worse as we age, especially when we're feeling tired or fed up, can mean that the mobility of this area starts to be restricted. Hunched walking posture can hamper our breathing as well as making us look and feel older than our years, so it definitely needs correcting. This exercise will help open out the chest area and strengthen the upper back (see thoracic spine, page 30), so that as you age your posture remains upright and strong. If you're not sure about the suitability of this exercise, begin with the Starter Pack version on page 76 and when you're comfortable with it, move on to this version where you lift your arms off the floor. Once confident with that, you can advance to completing more repetitions.

ALL LEVELS

Method

- Lie down on your front.
- Place a block or small cushion under your forehead – this is to keep your neck and spine aligned.
- Bend your arms so that your elbows are level with your shoulders and resting on the floor.
- Take your legs a hip-distance apart with your toes slightly turned in.

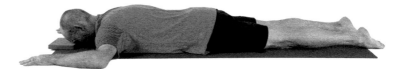

- Engage your abdominal muscles/pelvic floor muscles.
- Breathe in to your ribcage to prepare.
- Breathe out as you gently lift your head, your chest, your arms and elbows off the floor.
- Breathe in at the top.

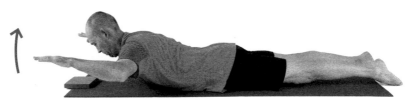

- Breathe out as you lower yourself slowly back to the floor.
- Repeat up to 6 times in total.

Too challenging? Try this:
- Return to the Starter Pack and begin with the Swan Dive on Forearms (page 76).

Not challenging enough? Try this:
- Perform more repetitions or hold for longer in the lifted position.

- Follow with Cat Stretch (page 77) to lengthen your spine in the opposite direction.

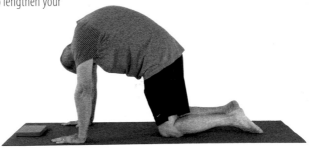

Note:
- Keep your neck and spine aligned, lengthening through your neck as you raise your head.
- Try to keep the movement flowing and not jerky.
- Your legs and glutes will want to help you; try your best to keep them relaxed and heavy – this takes practice, so be patient!

- Concentrate on your breathing and stay centred, pulling your abdomen up off the floor and engaging it throughout the exercise.
- If you get cramp (and some people do when their feet are turned in or in the pointed position), just curl your toes underneath and hopefully that will relieve the discomfort.

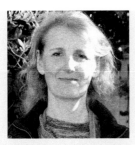

CASE STUDY

Deanne Ashman
Age: 50
Occupation: Chef
Favourite exercise: Swan Dive – I know it's good for my back!
Practised Pilates for: 3 years

'I started Pilates because of persistent lower backache and now I'm able to do more physically and no longer take painkillers. I know people with chronic back pain who have waited months to be seen on the NHS and are taking a cocktail of painkillers – Pilates is non-invasive and drug free. Before I did Pilates, I would often have lower backache, but Pilates has taken this away – core strength and regular movement is a definite cure.'

LEG PULL/PLANK

Benefits

This is a version of the well-known Plank exercise which encourages pelvic and shoulder stabilization while strengthening all the core muscles, and of course your arms. It also stretches the front of the hips and calf muscles. The Leg Pull/Planks are very powerful and will improve your overall general stamina and stability. These include Side Plank (page 117) and Reverse Leg Pull/Plank (page 155).

Note: if you have weak wrists, a shoulder injury, have had recent breast surgery or find your abdominal muscles aren't quite strong enough, just stick to the beginner version remaining on your knees. But if your knees are a little uncomfortable, put a cushion under each one to take some pressure off – the same applies to your elbows.

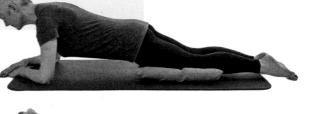

BEGINNER

Method

- Lie on your front and come up on to your forearms – elbows directly below your shoulders.

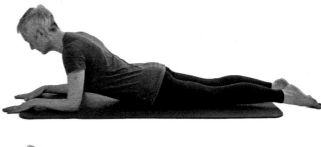

- Engage your abdominal muscles/ pelvic floor muscles.
- Breathe in to prepare.
- Breathe out as you lift your pelvis a little way and come on to your knees, feeling your abdominal muscles contract as you do so.

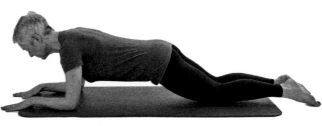

- Breathe in through your nose and into your ribcage and out through your mouth – continue using your lateral thoracic breathing (page 39) to help you concentrate and maintain the position.
- Make sure you keep your neck and spine aligned and that your abdominal muscles/pelvic floor muscles stay engaged.

- If you start to feel tension in your back, then stop, come down on to the floor, rest for a second or two and try again – you should feel the abdominal muscles working.
- Hold for up to 10 seconds to start with (or however long you can manage) and then start to increase the time as you feel stronger – aim for 30 seconds if you can!
- When you've completed the exercise sit back on your heels in Extended Child's Pose.

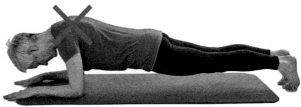

INTERMEDIATE
Method
- Lie on your front and come up on to your forearms – elbows placed directly below your shoulders.

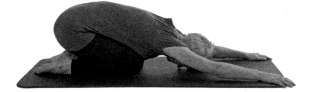

- Engage your abdominal muscles/ pelvic floor muscles.
- Breathe in to prepare.
- Breathe out and lift yourself up into a straight line and on to the balls of your feet.

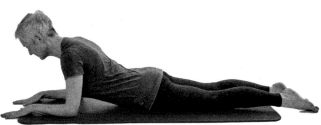

- Stabilize in that position and concentrate on breathing – in through your nose and in to your ribcage and then out through your mouth, for a total of 4 breaths.
- Keep your legs lengthened and feet on the floor.
- Maintain your neck and spine alignment throughout – don't drop your head down or tilt it upwards.

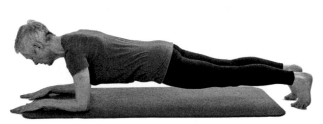

Note:

- Once in the intermediate Leg Pull/Plank position, there should be a straight line from your feet to your head.
- Stay in this Neutral Spine position.
- Make sure your back doesn't sag or your bottom lift up – remember you are a plank!

- Keep your abdominal muscles activated throughout.
- Focus on your breathing as it will help with concentration.

ADVANCED

Only attempt this exercise if you are confident with the other versions.

Method

- Start this advanced level Leg Pull/Plank exercise on your hands and knees.
- Make sure your hands/arms are directly under your shoulders.
- Keep your neck and spine aligned.
- Slide one leg directly behind you and come on to the ball of the foot.

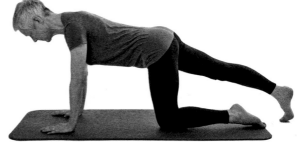

- Repeat on the other side until you are in the Leg Pull/Plank position.

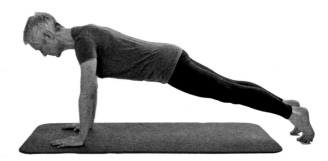

- Engage your abdominal muscles/pelvic floor muscles.
- Breathe in to prepare.
- Breathe out and lift one leg off the floor, simultaneously pushing the heel of the other foot down towards the floor.

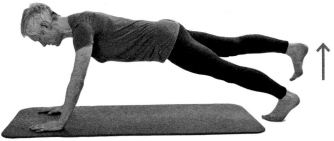

- Breathe in and hold.
- Breathe out and lower the leg back down into the start position.
- Repeat on the other side.
- Repeat the leg movement, alternating up to 6 times.
- At the end of the exercise come into Extended Child's Pose.

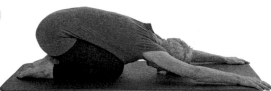

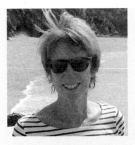

CASE STUDY

Sarah Hill
Age: 63
Practised Pilates for: 15 years
Favourite exercise: Plank (page 89)

'I started Pilates as part of my preparation for running the London Marathon. Now I have better core strength and balance for tennis and skiing. I used to have back problems but since doing Pilates regularly I haven't had any. I'm more upright now too and physically stronger, more confident in my ability to carry objects, climb stairs, etc. I used to feel I had a weak body. Not any more!'

SUPERMAN

Benefits

This exercise trains you to keep your torso stable while you move your arms and legs, which is exactly what we want to happen when we move about in daily life or play sport. It encourages good coordination and strengthens and lengthens the spinal extensor (erector spinae) muscles which support the spine. This improves walking posture while building stability in the core and shoulder muscles.

> ***Note:*** *if you find it uncomfortable to kneel on the floor or you have problems with your knees, either pad the knee area with a towel or cushion or choose the Swimming exercise (page 82) instead. The same applies to wrist problems, if you find it uncomfortable putting pressure on your wrists, either pad the area under your hands or choose the Swimming exercise instead. Take advice if you've recently had breast surgery.*

BEGINNER

Method

- Start on all fours, knees directly under hips, arms directly below your shoulders.
- Keep your neck and spine aligned, with your eyes focused on the floor.

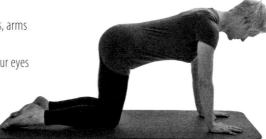

- Engage your abdominal muscles/pelvic floor muscles.
- Breathe in to prepare.
- Breathe out through your mouth and slowly slide one foot directly behind you on the floor, toes pointed.
- Breathe in as you hold the lengthened position.
- Breathe out as you slide the leg back into position.
- Repeat on the other side and then complete up to 8 repetitions in total.

INTERMEDIATE

Method

- Start on all fours, knees directly under hips, arms directly below your shoulders.
- Keep your neck and spine aligned, with your eyes focused on the floor.

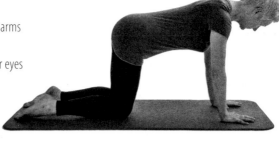

- Engage your abdominal muscles/pelvic floor muscles.
- Breathe in to prepare.
- Breathe out through your mouth and slowly slide your foot directly behind you on the floor, toes pointed.
- Breathe in and hold the position.

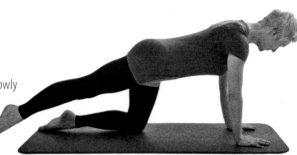

- Breathe out and raise the leg to hip height.
- Breathe in again and hold the position, being aware of your pelvic stability.

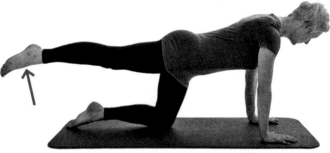

- Breathe out and lower the leg down to the floor, keeping it lengthened, and then slide back into position.
- Repeat on the other side and then complete up to 8 repetitions in total.

ADVANCED

Method

- As for the Beginners and Intermediate versions, start on all fours, knees directly under hips, arms under your shoulders.
- Keep your neck and spine aligned, with your eyes focused on the floor.

- Engage your abdominal muscles/pelvic floor muscles.
- Breathe in to prepare.
- Breathe out through your mouth and slowly slide one foot directly behind you on the floor, toes pointed, while simultaneously beginning to extend your opposite arm up in front of you.

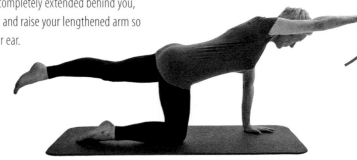

- When your leg is completely extended behind you, lift it to hip height and raise your lengthened arm so it is level with your ear.

- Balance and hold that position.
- Breathe in to your ribcage.
- Breathe out as you simultaneously lower both your arm and leg, with control, back down to the floor, sliding your leg back into position beside your other knee.
- Repeat on the other side.
- Repeat up to 10 times (5 on each side).

- After you've completed this exercise, come into Extended Child's Pose (page 78) so that any tensions are released. While in Extended Child's Pose, stretch your arms ahead of you and rotate your wrists if they're feeling a bit stiff.

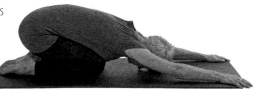

- Stay in that position for about 20 seconds. Then move your arms round by your sides to relieve any tension in your shoulders.

Note:

- Be aware of your pelvis particularly in the intermediate and advanced versions – is it dropping down on one side or shifting outwards as you lift your leg up to hip height?

- Aim to keep your torso as stable as possible – imagine you are balancing a tray of full champagne glasses on your back.
- Keep the exercise flowing, concentrate on your breathing and keep centred.

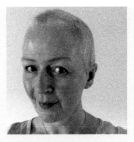

CASE STUDY

Fiona O'Donovan
Age: 49
Occupation: professional muddler-through!
Practised Pilates for: 2 years
Favourite exercises: Roll Down (page 51), balance exercises and Push-Up (page 104).

'I'm a runner and I was getting injured a lot. I took up Pilates as I want to keep running forever. You can't improve your balance by lifting weights or Zumba, you can only improve it by practising balance when you're standing up or lying down. Since taking up Pilates I haven't had sore knees, sore hips, sore ankles or a sore ITB. My pelvic floor muscles have also definitely strengthened, I've noticed a difference and that is so important as we age. When you're younger you can do so much with such ease but you don't realize that as you get older things change. It does come back quickly – but disappears quickly if you don't keep it up! I come out of class feeling better, lighter, happier – you don't have to be the fastest or the strongest. I come out feeling de-stressed.'

DART WITH TRICEP LIFT

Benefits

This exercise is primarily a back strengthener and mobilizer with the added bonus, in the intermediate and advanced versions, of some arm and shoulder work. It also encourages good walking and standing posture by extending the spine. If you're a power walker or use Nordic Walking poles, then strengthening your *triceps* (back of arms) and shoulders will prevent your arms from becoming tired while propelling yourself forwards.

BEGINNER

Method

- Lie on your front and place your forehead on a block or cushion.
  Take your arms down by your sides, palms turned up.
- Bring your big toes together
  and let your heels flop
  open to relax your legs.

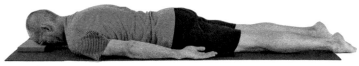

- Engage your abdominal muscles/pelvic floor muscles.
- Breathe in to prepare.
- As you breathe out, lift your
  head, chest and arms up off
  the floor.

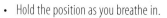

- Hold the position as you breathe in.
- Breathe out and slowly lower yourself back down to the floor.
- Repeat up to 6 times.

- Follow with Cat Stretch (page 77) to lengthen your
  spine in the opposite direction.

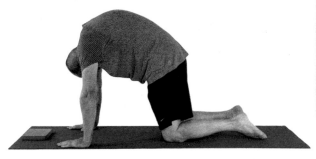

Note:
- Make sure you are keeping your neck and spine aligned – look down, rather than tilting your head upwards.
- Remember to lengthen the neck – it sometimes gets forgotten!
- Avoid tensing your shoulders, and keep your abdominal muscles engaged throughout.
- Concentrate on your breathing to help the exercise flow.

INTERMEDIATE

Method

- Engage your abdominal muscles/pelvic floor muscles.
- Breathe in to prepare.
- As you breathe out, lift your head, chest and arms up off the floor.

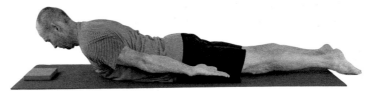

- Using short out breaths, pulse your arms upwards from the shoulders for the count of up to 10.

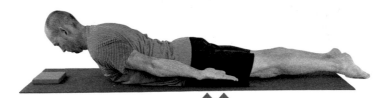

- On completion of the 10 pulses, hold the position.

- Breathe in to your ribcage again.
- Breathe out through your mouth as you return your chest and arms back to the floor.
- Repeat up to 8 times in total.
- Follow with Cat Stretch to lengthen your spine in the opposite direction.

ADVANCED

- Increase the repetitions.
- Use hand weights. But make sure that if you do, you keep your neck lengthened and your legs relaxed. Don't let the hand weights alter the alignment of your body.

ROTATIONAL CAT

Benefits

This exercise will strengthen your core muscles and challenge your balance. It will also increase flexibility throughout the whole of your back as it rotates your spine and will open out and stretch your chest muscles. The thoracic spine (page 30) can become stiff and excessively curved as we age, and this exercise will encourage good posture which over time will go some way to preventing the curvature. This is also a great exercise for the day after a long walk or a lot of activity, to balance the body after a golf or tennis session, for example, especially if you tend to suffer from backache. If you sit slouched over a desk all day, you'll find the rotational movement of the exercise relieves the postural tension that this can cause.

Note: if it's uncomfortable to kneel on the floor, place a rolled-up towel or cushion underneath each knee for more comfort. If you have wrist or elbow problems, you might want to omit this exercise or put some padding under the hand/wrist that has pressure on it. If you have any serious back problems, please consult your medical practitioner before attempting the exercise to make sure that a rotational exercise is suitable for your condition.

BEGINNER/INTERMEDIATE

Method

- Start the exercise on your hands and knees.
- Place your hands directly under your shoulders, knees under your hips.
- Keep your head and spine aligned.

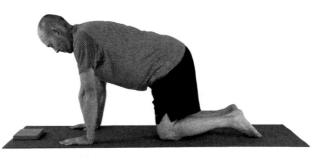

- Engage your abdominal muscles/ pelvic floor muscles.
- Breathe in to prepare.
- Breathe out and take your right arm off the ground and thread it between your left arm and left leg.

- Bend your left elbow.

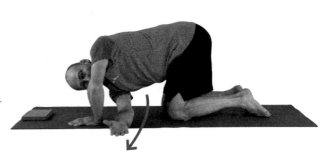

- Lower your head and right shoulder down to the mat for a deeper rotation as long as you are comfortable to do so.

- Breathe in and hold the rotational stretch.
- Breathe out and rotate back the other way, taking your right arm up in the air, this time following it with your head and neck.

- Breathe in at the top as you hold the position.
- Breathe out as you return to the mat.
- Continue rotating, keeping the exercise flowing from side to side.

- Repeat up to 6 times, and then come down into Extended Child's pose (page 78) to give your wrist a rest before changing sides.

Want more of a challenge? Try this:
- Increase repetitions.

Note:
- Don't force the rotation; only go as far as you are comfortable especially if you are very stiff or have back issues.
- Keep your abdominal muscles engaged throughout to support your spine.
- Let the exercise flow and concentrate on your breathing – take care not to hold your breath.

SINGLE LEG KICK

Benefits

This exercise will give your quads (front of thighs) and hip flexors a good stretch. When you're walking or jogging the hip flexors work hard, repeatedly raising your leg: they contract and then shorten each time. So if they become tight, your pelvis can begin to tilt forwards and this can lead to backache. The Single Leg Kick will also strengthen the glutes (buttocks), hamstrings (back of thighs), upper arms and back. The glutes can often be a problem for anyone who jogs or power walks, either because they're not firing properly or are weak — often the cause of lumbar and pelvic instability — as discussed in Chapter 5.

BEGINNER

Note: *if you have knee problems, please take a look at the suggested modifications at the end of the exercise.*

Method

- Lie on your front.
- Come on to your forearms, elbows sitting just below your shoulders.
- Make fists with your hands.

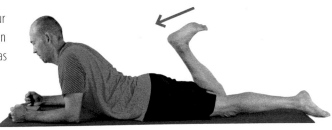

- Engage your abdominal muscles/pelvic floor muscles.
- Breathe in to your ribcage to prepare.
- Breathe out and kick one heel towards your buttock, pulsing twice.

- Lengthen and extend the leg back out along the floor as you breathe in again.
- Breathe out and repeat with your other leg, pulsing twice and then extending back along the floor as you breathe in.

• Repeat up to 8 times as long as you are comfortable, alternating legs, and then come into Cat Stretch (page 77).

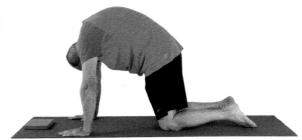

Note:
• Make sure you keep your abdominal muscles engaged throughout the exercise.
• Be aware of any arching in your back and your general alignment.
• Concentrate on your breathing to help the exercise flow more easily.

Knee problems? Try this:
• Rather than kicking, keep the movement smooth and move the leg only in a comfortable range; don't pulse. Or omit the exercise altogether.

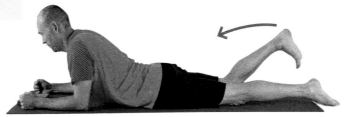

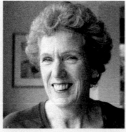

CASE STUDY

Jilli Williams
Age: 65
Occupation: Graphic designer
Practised Pilates for: 10 years
Favourite exercise: Roll Down (page 51)

'Curiosity took me to Pilates. Now I find my breathing and my balance are better when playing tennis. I am more flexible through the stretching and I can lift heavy weights with confidence now I use my tummy muscles to support my back. When I walk I now remember to look forwards and not down at the floor, stretching to my full height. Also through practise I'm aware of not moving too fast when bending down and lifting things, more aware of what my body can do – I can stretch and bend further than before.'

DOUBLE LEG KICK

Benefits

This exercise is a progression of Single Leg Kick (page 100), so make sure you are comfortable with that exercise before attempting this one. The Double Leg Kick generates the same benefits as Single Leg Kick, but is more challenging. It strengthens the glutes (buttocks), hip flexors and back muscles while stretching the front of the thighs and opening out the chest. It also challenges stability and improves coordination – both of which we need to work on as we age in order to keep on doing what we've always loved!

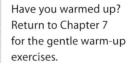

Have you warmed up? Return to Chapter 7 for the gentle warm-up exercises.

Note: *if you have knee problems, please take a look at the modifications towards the end of the exercise and adapt accordingly.*

INTERMEDIATE

Method

- Lie on your front.
- Turn your head to one side.
- Move both hands to your lower back and clasp them together resting there.
- Let your elbows sink towards the floor at the side of your torso.
- Bring your extended legs together and point your toes.

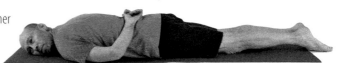

- Engage your abdominal muscles/ pelvic floor muscles.
- Breathe in to your ribcage to prepare.
- Breathe out as you bend your knees and kick both heels towards your buttocks, pulsing three times.

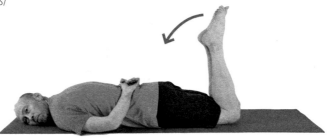

- Breathe in as you lengthen the legs back along the mat.
- Breathe out as you lift your chest off the floor, straightening your arms, hands still clasped along your back, simultaneously lifting your legs and lengthening them away from you.

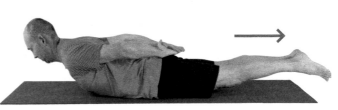

- Breathe in, lower the legs and your torso back down to the floor, turning your head to face the other direction.
- Breathe out and relax.
- Repeat up to 6 times in total, then come into Cat Stretch (page 77).

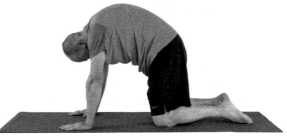

Note:
- To begin with you may find it easier to breathe naturally and perform this exercise with more speed.
- Keep your legs lengthened together.
- Keep your hips glued to the mat as you kick your heels back.

Knee problems or stiff shoulders? Try these:
- Perform the exercise slowly within a comfortable range of movement.
- Perform Single Leg Kick (page 100).

- If your shoulders are stiff, leave your arms down by your sides and just perform the leg movements.

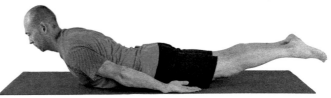

ADVANCED

- Increase the repetitions.
- Reach your clasped hands further down your back and lift your torso higher.
- Make sure you open up your chest rather than straining from your lower back.

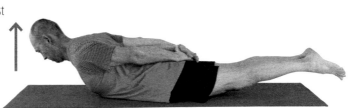

PUSH-UP FROM STANDING

Benefits

This can be a challenging exercise, so not for the beginner. But it is an excellent strengthening exercise for the arms (especially the triceps at the back of your upper arm) and pectoral (chest) muscles. It encourages good shoulder stability, core strength and spinal mobility. It also works on your stamina and balance. Over time this will improve your posture. In addition this exercise will lengthen your hamstrings and quads.

INTERMEDIATE

Method

- Stand tall, lengthening through your spine.
- Engage your abdominal muscles/pelvic floor muscles.
- Breathe in to prepare.
- Breathe out and slowly roll down towards your mat (see Roll Down, page 51) with your legs straight (as long as this is comfortable) until your hands reach or nearly reach the ground – don't worry if this isn't possible, just go as far as you can.

- Breathe in.
- Breathe out and walk your hands forwards, bending your knees if you need to, keeping your heels down and legs straight.

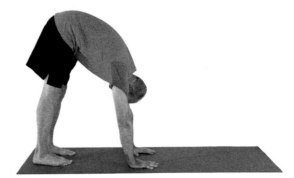

- Breathing naturally, come down into the Leg Pull/Plank position (page 88), hands aligned under your shoulders.

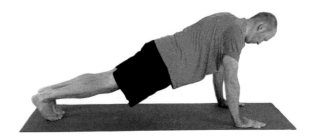

- Bend your knees down on to the floor.
- Cross your ankles and bring your heels up behind your buttocks.

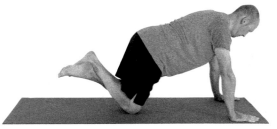
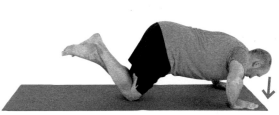

- Breathe in as you bend your elbows and take your torso down towards the mat. Make sure the body moves as one, rather than dipping at the hips and arching the back.

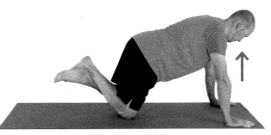

- Breathe out as you push up.

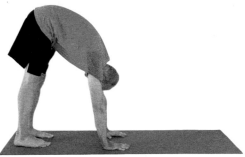

- Repeat 3 push-ups in total.
- Breathe in and push your hips up towards the ceiling.
- Breathe out and walk your hands back towards your feet.
- Breathe in and hold the position.
- Breathe out and slowly uncurl back up to standing, making sure your abdominal muscles are engaged as you do so.
- Repeat up to 3 times.

Too challenging? Try this:
- Move your hands slightly wider than your shoulders before you perform the push-up.

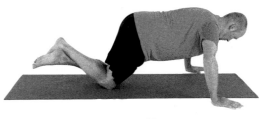

- Keep the push-up small until you feel stronger – just take your torso a little way towards the floor.

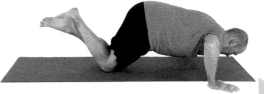

ADVANCED

Note: please only attempt this if you are strong enough and can complete the Intermediate version comfortably. This version of the exercise strengthens the triceps even more.

Method

- Stand tall, lengthening through your spine into Neutral Spine position.
- Engage your abdominal muscles/pelvic floor muscles.
- Breathe in to prepare.
- Breathe out and slowly roll down towards your mat with your legs straight until your hands reach or nearly reach the ground. If you have tight hamstrings, bend your knees to bring yourself closer to the floor so that you can take the weight on to your hands.

- Breathe in.
- Breathe out and walk your hands forwards, keeping your heels down on the floor, or as near to the floor as possible and legs straight.

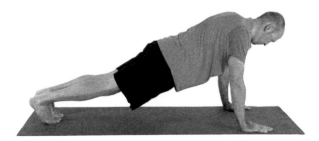

- Breathing naturally, come down into the Leg Pull/Plank position (page 88), hands aligned under your shoulders.

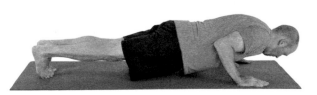

- Breathe in and lower yourself slowly towards the floor, keeping your elbows close to your ribs as they bend.

- Breathe out and push up back into the Plank position.

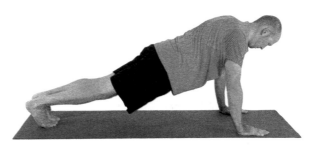

- Repeat up to 3 push-ups in total.
- Breathe in and push your hips up towards the ceiling.
- Breathe out and walk your hands back towards your feet.
- Hold the position as you breathe in.

- Breathe out and slowly uncurl back up to standing, remembering to keep your abdominal muscles engaged.

- Repeat up to 6 times, each time performing 3 push-ups.

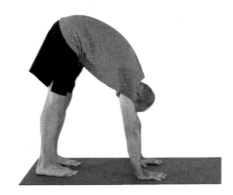

- Keep your abdominal muscles engaged throughout.
- Concentrate on your breathing and keep the movement slow and controlled.
- Maintain Neutral Spine throughout.

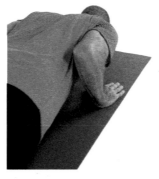

Note:
- Don't be tempted to move your hands forwards, keep them aligned under the shoulders.
- Try and stroke your ribs with your elbows as you lower yourself to the ground.

Too challenging?
- Perform Push-Up from Standing (intermediate) (page 104).
- Perform fewer repetitions.
- Keep the push-up small, only go a little way until you feel stronger.

CAT STRETCH INTO DOWN DOG

Benefits

A great exercise to lengthen the hamstrings, calf muscles and Achilles tendons either after activity or during an exercise routine. It also strengthens the upper body and spine and develops your coordination skills – a great combination of yoga and Pilates.

ALL LEVELS

Method

- Start on all fours in a neutral position.
- Make sure your arms are aligned under your shoulders and your knees under your hips.

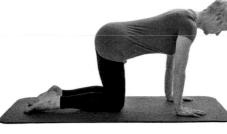

- Engage your abdominal muscles/pelvic floor muscles.
- Breathe in to prepare.
- Breathe out as you lengthen through your spine and arch into Cat Stretch (page 77).

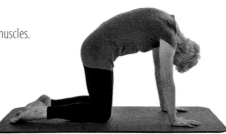

- Curl your toes under, drop your head and lift your knees.
- Breathe in as you send your spine up into the air, your tailbone towards the ceiling.

- Breathe out as you lengthen your calf muscles and gently ease your heels down towards the floor.
- Breathe in and hold the calf stretch.

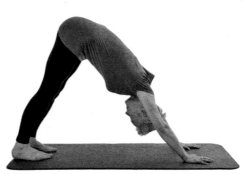

- Breathe out and come on to the balls of your feet, keeping your head dropped and your arms straight.
- Breathe in and hold the position.

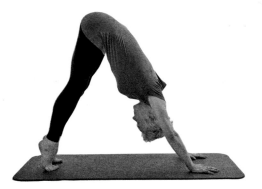

- Breathe out as you push your heels back down into the floor.
- Breathe in and hold that stretch.

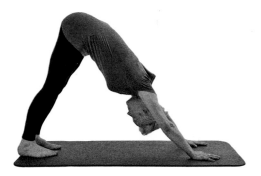

- Breathe out and repeat the foot movements for up to 4 repetitions in total.
- Come back down on to your hands and knees and into Extended Child's Pose (page 78).

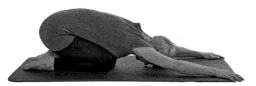

Note:
- Keep your weight evenly distributed between your feet and arms.
- Try not to tense your shoulders.
- If you find the breathing sequence too fast, just adapt accordingly.

Too challenging? Try this:
- Bend your knees if you find the stretch in the legs too intense. If you struggle to lengthen the spine fully with the legs straight, soften the knees and send the tailbone higher, to make sure the upper back isn't rounded but you are more in an inverted 'V' shape.

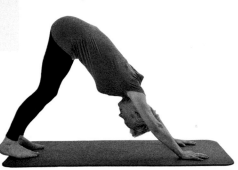

SIDE SERIES

So-called because the exercises are performed on your side. Remember to do both sides of your body — you'll be amazed at how one side feels different to the other, highlighting our postural imbalances. If you find it uncomfortable to lie on your side because your hips dig into the floor or mat, place a small towel under the area to make yourself more comfortable.

Side Kicks

Benefits

All of the following Side Kick exercises work on your core muscles, specifically your oblique (waist) muscles and hip area. The stronger the oblique muscles, the less likelihood of pelvis and hip problems particularly if you're sedentary and so more at risk due to lack of strength. You'll also find that these exercises strengthen and lengthen the *tensor fasciae latae* (TFL) and *iliotibial band* (ITB). The TFL sits at the top of the ITB to the front, by the side of your hip and the ITB is the tendon that runs down the outside of your thigh to your knee. It helps to stabilize the knee and flexes, abducts (takes the leg out to the side) and rotates the hip joint, so if you jog or walk long distances you need to keep it happy!

SIDE KICK 1

BEGINNER/INTERMEDIATE

Method

- Lie on your side.
- Lengthen your underneath arm directly under your head.
- Place your head on a block or small cushion which you can balance on your upper arm. This will keep your neck and spine aligned.

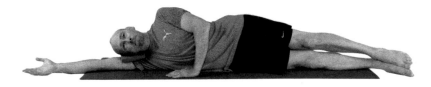

- Glance down towards your feet, check that your hips, knees and ankles are stacked and aligned.
- Place your other hand in front of your torso on the floor for support.
- Engage your abdominal muscles/pelvic floor muscles.

- Breathe in to prepare.
- As you breathe out, raise both legs together in a straight line off the floor. They don't have to go very high, just a little way and no higher than your hips.

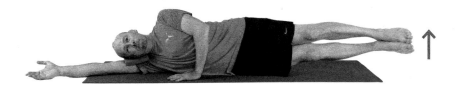

- Breathe in and hold the raised position.
- As you breathe out, slowly lower the legs, with control, down to the floor.
- Repeat up to 10 times.
- Turn over and perform the exercise on the other side.

Too challenging? Try this:
- Return to Starter Pack (page 68) and perform the Single Leg version.

ADVANCED

- Use ankle weights on one or both legs, but make sure you keep them lengthened and aligned during the exercise.
- Increase repetitions as you become more comfortable with the exercise.

Note:
- Try not to push your supporting hand down into the floor. Imagine you're resting it on the surface of water: keep the arm and shoulder relaxed.
- Concentrate on your breathing to keep the movements flowing and to avoid any jerky actions.

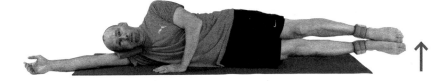

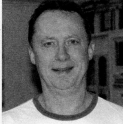

CASE STUDY

Phil Pask
Age: 51
Occupation: Managing Director
Practised Pilates for: 3 years
Favourite exercise: Roll Down (page 51)

'I started Pilates because I want to remain supple and to keep going for as long as possible. My work involves a lot of driving and Pilates counteracts all the sitting I do. I certainly feel stronger for it and I've noticed that my posture has improved. As part of my work I lift heavy things in and out of vans and I've never had a bad back or any other niggles – I really think this is because I have a greater consciousness, through Pilates, about engaging my core when lifting. As I get older I appreciate the importance of looking after my body, keeping flexible, fit and healthy and Pilates definitely helps.'

SIDE KICK 2 + INNER THIGH

For benefits, see page 110.

Have you warmed up?
Return to Chapter 7
for the gentle warm-up
exercises.

BEGINNER/INTERMEDIATE
Method

- Lie on your side.
- Lengthen your underneath arm directly under your head. Place your head on a block or small cushion balanced between the upper part of your arm and your head.

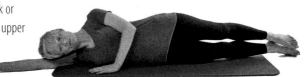

- Glance down towards your feet, check that your hips, knees and ankles are stacked and aligned.
- Place your other hand in front of your torso on the floor for support.
- Engage your abdominal muscles/pelvic floor muscles.
- Breathe in to prepare.
- As you breathe out, raise both legs together in a straight line off the floor.

- Breathe in and hold the raised position.
- Breathe out and lift the top leg higher.

- Breathe in and hold the position.
- Breathe out and lower the top leg down to join the lower leg.

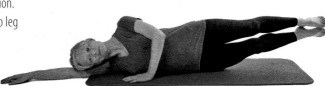

- Return both legs to floor.
- Repeat up to 10 times and continue with the following Inner Thigh exercise before turning over and performing the exercise on the other side.

INNER THIGH

- Engage your abdominal muscles/pelvic floor muscles.
- Place your supporting hand in front of you and keep your arm relaxed.
- Breathe in to prepare.
- Breathe out and raise both legs together in a straight line off the floor.
- Point your toes.

- Breathe in and hold the position.
- Breathe out and raise your top leg slightly higher.

- Breathe in and hold the position.
- Breathe out and lift your lower leg up to meet the leg above.

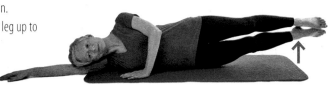

- Breathing naturally, continue to lift and lower the underneath leg for up to 10 repetitions.

Too challenging? Try this:

- Return to the Starter Pack and perform Single Leg Side Kick (page 75) until you feel ready to progress.

Note:

- If you find the breathing challenging, just concentrate on engaging your abdominals and balancing to begin with. Breathe naturally until you get into a rhythm.
- Try not to press the supporting hand down in front of your torso – keep the body relaxed.
- Be aware of what your shoulders are doing. Keep them stabilized – make sure they're not rising up around your ears.

ADVANCED

- Perform more repetitions.
- Use ankle weights on both ankles or just the lower leg that is working the inner thigh.
- Put your supporting hand on to your upper thigh, challenging your balance further.

SIDE KICK 3 INTO TORPEDO

Benefits

The same benefits as before (page 110), but the Torpedo encourages and improves torso stability even more because of the arm extension – so if you feel a bit wobbly to start with, persevere and it will get easier.

INTERMEDIATE

Method

- Lie on your side.
- Lengthen your underneath arm directly under your head. Place your head on a block or small cushion which you can balance on the upper part of your arm.

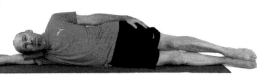

- Glance down towards your feet, check that your hips, knees and ankles are stacked and aligned.
- Engage your abdominal muscles/pelvic floor muscles.
- Take your other hand and rest it, lengthening your arm as you do so, along your top thigh.

- Breathe in to prepare.
- Breathe out as you simultaneously raise both legs and extend your top arm over your head into the Torpedo position.

- Point your toes.
- Hold the position as you breathe in.
- Breathe out as you return your legs and arm to the starting position.
- Repeat up to 10 times on each side or perform as many repetitions as you feel comfortable.

Note:
- Focus on lengthening your legs and arms, reaching out from a strong centre and keeping your abdominal muscles engaged.
- Use your breathing to help the exercise flow and try to avoid any jerky body movements.
- Balancing with the arm extended can be challenging – keep practising and it will become easier as your balance improves.

ADVANCED

- Hold a small hand weight as you extend your arm over your head and/or use ankle weights on your legs. But make sure you can still perform the exercise well, keeping the torso aligned and stable.

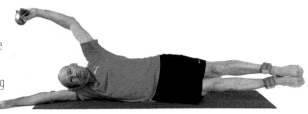

SIDE BEND

Benefits

The Side Bend, or Side Plank as it's sometimes known, challenges your core stability and over time will improve your strength and stamina – useful as we age. As with the previous Side Kick exercises you'll find your oblique (waist) muscles working hard; this exercise will strengthen the muscles and so prevent unnecessary twisting when walking or jogging. The Side Bend also works the shoulders, the supporting arm and improves hip mobility.

BEGINNER

Method

- Sit on your right buttock, leaning on your elbow.

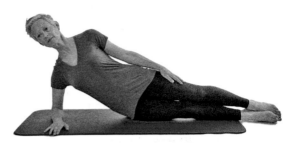

- Bend both knees to your side, heels in line with your torso.
- Bring your left foot to the front of your right foot.
- Keep your knees bent to your side throughout the exercise.
- Take your left hand and rest on your top leg, keeping the arm relaxed.

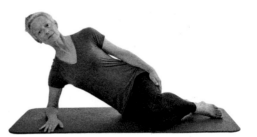

- Engage your abdominal muscles/ pelvic floor muscles.
- Breathe in to prepare.
- Breathe out as you lift your pelvis off the floor from the bent knee position.
- Breathe in and hold the position.

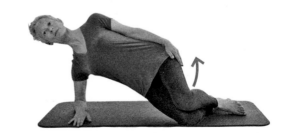

- Breathe out and lower yourself back down to the floor.
- Repeat up to 4 times just raising and lowering the pelvis before including the arm in the exercise.
- The next time, when you raise your pelvis up, simultaneously lengthen your top arm over your head.

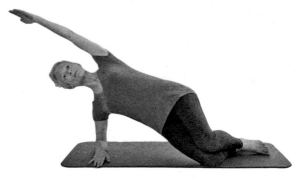

- Breathe in at the top.
- Breathe out as you return to the start position.
- Repeat up to 4 times.
- Repeat the exercise on the other side.

INTERMEDIATE/ADVANCED

Method

- Sit on your right buttock, leaning on your right arm/hand.
- Place your hand flat on the floor, slightly wider than your shoulder.
- Bend both knees to your side, heels in line with your torso.
- Bring your left foot to the front of your right foot.

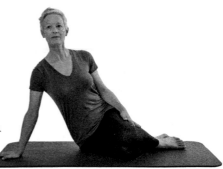

- Take your left arm and rest it on your left thigh, palm up.
- Engage your abdominal muscles/ pelvic floor muscles.
- Keep your chest open and lengthen through your spine.
- Breathe in to prepare.
- Breathe out and extend your legs away from you in a straight line as you raise up your pelvis and reach your top arm over your head into the Side Bend position.

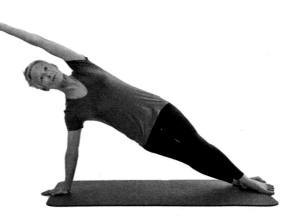

- Breathe in again as you balance and hold the pose.
- Breathe out, bend both knees as you lower yourself slowly, with control, back to the floor, bringing your top arm down to rest at the same time.
- Repeat up to 4 times each side.

Note:

- Try not to let your hips sag or drop down: keep them lifted, stable and facing forwards.
- Keep your abdominal muscles engaged throughout.
- Concentrate on your breathing and lengthening through your legs and arm as you perform the exercise.

CLAM

Benefits

This exercise (also known as Lateral Hip Opener) is a must for everyone. It targets your gluteus medius muscle, the middle-sized buttock muscle that works to encourage pelvic and knee stability. If this muscle becomes tight or shortened the pelvic instability it causes can lead to lower backache, knee and hip problems. It's also an excellent exercise for the Iliotibial band and the Tensor Fasciae Latae (see page 110 for information about the ITB tendon and the TFL) because it lengthens them both along with the hip rotators. In addition, the Clam can often help with sciatic pain and hamstring strain.

BEGINNER/INTERMEDIATE

Method

- Lie on your side.
- Lengthen your underneath arm directly under your head and place your head on a block or small cushion on the upper part of your arm.
- Bend both knees and keep your heels in line with your buttocks.

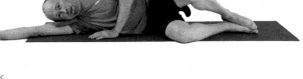

- Engage your abdominal muscles/pelvic floor muscles.
- Breathe naturally.
- Raise your top knee just a small amount, keeping your feet on the floor.

- Return your knee to the starting position.
- Repeat up to 16 times and then change sides.

ADVANCED

- Lift your feet off the floor, keeping your heels in line with your bottom.

- Repeat the same knee-opening movement in this position, making sure you maintain pelvic stability. Imagine your pelvis is resting against a wall: turn your thigh bone like a key in a lock, just a small movement to activate the gluteus medius muscle.
- Repeat up to 10 times.
- On the last repetition hold the knee open and gently pulse the knee upwards 10 times.
- Change sides and repeat.

Note:
- Keep your feet glued together throughout and your torso stable.
- If you feel your pelvis rotating (moving) backwards, you are opening up your knee too far. Keep the movement small so the pelvis remains upright.

OUTER AND INNER THIGH LIFTS

OUTER THIGH LIFT (ABDUCTOR MUSCLES)

Benefits

This is not a classic Pilates exercise but one well worth including in a book on Pilates for living. This exercise will not only strengthen the outer thigh, ITB (see page 110) and glutes but also improve your walking form and posture. The *quadriceps* are the muscles at the front of the thigh which help keep the kneecap stable. This exercise, like all the side-lying exercises, also challenges balance and strengthens the core muscles.

BEGINNER/INTERMEDIATE

Method

- Lie on your side.
- Lengthen your underneath arm directly under your head and place your head on a block or small cushion on the upper part of your arm.
- Place your other hand in front of you on the floor for support.
- Check that you are in Neutral Spine and make sure your body is in a straight line, hips, knees and ankles stacked.
- Bend your underneath leg in front of you.
- Lengthen your top leg, rotating your foot so that your toes face forwards.

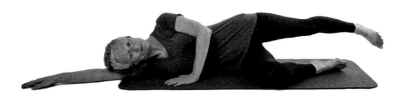

- Engage your abdominal muscles/pelvic floor muscles.
- Breathe in to your ribcage to prepare.
- Breathe out and raise your top leg, keeping it lengthened.

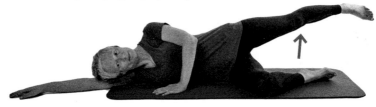

- Breathe in at the top and then as you lower your leg back down, breathe out.
- Repeat up to 16 times in total, or aim for a few to start with and increase the repetitions when you feel stronger. Follow it with the Inner Thigh Lift (page 113).

Note:
- Be aware of your pelvic stability – make sure there is no wobble. If there is, don't take your leg so high.
- Relax your shoulders and your supporting arm; try not to take any tension in the upper body.
- Concentrate on your breathing to help the exercise flow and avoid jerky movements.
- Keep your abdominal muscles engaged throughout.

ADVANCED
- Increase repetitions.
- Take your supporting arm and lengthen it along your top thigh as you lift. This will challenge your balance.
- Use ankle weights as long as you can keep your body aligned.

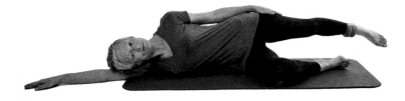

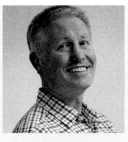

CASE STUDY
Gareth Jones
Age: 53
Occupation: Manager
Practised Pilates for: 1 year
Favourite exercise: Rotational Cat – I perform it 3 or 4 times a week (page 98)

'I've always stretched and previously I've done yoga but the benefits I find from Pilates are mental sharpness, confidence and increased wellbeing. I walk, jog and cycle and my lower back and stomach muscles are stronger – I think it's great for improving posture, flexibility and general fitness.'

INNER THIGH LIFT (ADDUCTOR MUSCLES)

Benefits

This exercise accompanies the Outer Thigh Lift (page 120) and it's important to practise them together. The benefits are the same, although this exercise will strengthen the adductor muscles (inner thigh) and increase pelvic stability.

Have you warmed up? Return to Chapter 7 for the gentle warm-up exercises.

BEGINNER/INTERMEDIATE

Method

- Lie on your side.
- Lengthen your underneath arm directly under your head and place your head on a block or small cushion which you can balance on the upper part of your arm.
- Place your other hand in front of you on the floor for support.
- Check that you are in Neutral Spine and make sure your body is in a straight line, hips, knees and ankles stacked.
- Bend your top leg and move your knee on to the floor in front of you.
- Lengthen your underneath leg and point your toes.

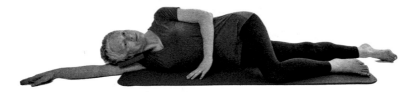

- Engage your abdominal muscles/pelvic floor muscles.
- Breathe in to prepare.
- Breathe out and raise your lower leg, lengthening it away, pointing your toes.

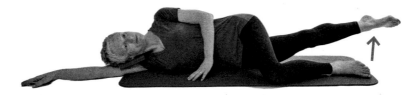

- Breathe in and lower your leg to hover above the floor; maintain the energy in the muscles, and try not to let them switch off.

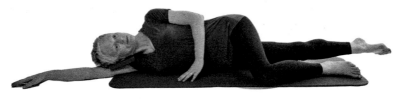

- Breathe out and lift again.
- Repeat up to 16 times in total or build up to this and start with less repetitions and then turn over and perform both this exercise and the Outer Thigh Lift (page 120) on the other side.
- Relax your shoulders and your supporting arm; try not to take any tension in the upper body.
- Keep your abdominal muscles engaged throughout.

ADVANCED

- Increase repetitions.
- Use ankle weights as long as you can keep your body aligned.

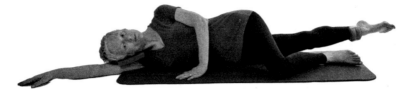

Note:
- Be aware of pelvic stability – if you find that your pelvis rolls forwards because your top leg is pulling it towards the floor, place a cushion underneath your front knee to raise it up.

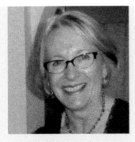

CASE STUDY

Carol Record
Age: 62
Occupation: Medical practitioner
Practised Pilates for: 3 years
Favourite exercise: Roll Down (page 51)

'I started Pilates because I needed to improve my core stability and my posture and balance. I've found that my back is more flexible and I get less sacroiliac (joints at the back of the pelvis) discomfort. It's a great way to start my day – I feel more energized and more confident that I won't experience back problems as I get older.'

CHEST OPENER

Benefits

This exercise can be performed either as a stretch on its own or during your regular Pilates session. It opens out the chest, stretching your pectoral muscles, which can become tight as your shoulders hunch forwards. Having an open chest means your lungs can work more efficiently. As you rotate in this exercise you'll be improving the mobility of your thoracic spine (page 30), strengthening the back muscles. Your shoulders and neck will also get a good stretch, releasing any tension or niggles that might be lurking and will help improve your posture.

ALL LEVELS

Method

- Lie on your side with knees bent and your heels in line with your buttocks.
- Place a block or small cushion under your head.
- Lengthen your underneath arm straight along the floor in front of your chest, palm up.
- Bring your other arm to rest on top of the lower arm, palms together.

- Engage your abdominal muscles/ pelvic floor muscles.
- Breathe in to prepare.
- Breathe out and raise your top arm up towards the ceiling, follow the movement with your gaze and begin to rotate your spine.

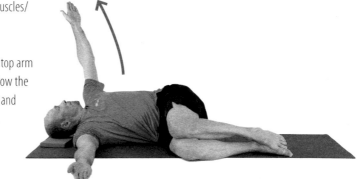

- Opening out from your chest and moving from your breastbone (rather than your arm), take your arm as far as your ribcage can comfortably twist, with your head, neck and spine following it.
- Breathe in as you hold the open rotation.
- Breathe out and return slowly to the start position.
- Repeat up to 6 times and then roll over to perform the exercise on the other side.

Note:

- Keep your hips stacked one on top of the other; don't let your pelvis rotate back with your spine, it needs to stay put.
- Your spine should rotate evenly, imagine your nose is in line with your breastbone: the shoulder blade stays softly aligned in the ribcage. If you feel it pinch, the arm has extended too far.

Too challenging? Try this:

- If the rotation is challenging and your chest muscles are very tight, just take your arm above and in line with your chest instead of rotating behind. Over time, as you work on your spinal mobility you will find that you'll be able to rotate further.

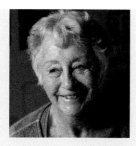

CASE STUDY

Patricia Woodhouse
Age: 81
Practised Pilates for: 1 year
Favourite exercise: any to do with balance

'Pilates was recommended to me by my physiotherapist after treatment for a knee problem and since doing Pilates my knees have definitely felt stronger. My stamina is improving and I'm learning to balance and walk better.'

FRONT SERIES

Take care: some of the exercises in the front series require forward flexion of the neck. If you suffer from any condition where this move might be contraindicated (osteoporosis or osteopaenia for example), please check the suitability of the exercise with your medical professional beforehand.

SINGLE KNEE FOLD

Benefits

This exercise teaches a very basic pelvic and torso stability. It is also a good hip mobility exercise and strengthens the lower back. Although this feels like a simple exercise, it relates well to any activity you might be doing – for example, when you are walking you are lifting alternate legs, just as you do in this exercise. The aim is to keep your torso stable while you're moving the leg, which is what we want to happen when we walk. While performing the exercise, pay special attention to what your pelvis is doing – does it lift up or shift? Keep those abdominal muscles engaged and you will notice a difference.

ALL LEVELS

Method

- Lie on your back with your knees bent and place your feet in line with your hips.
- Place a block or small cushion under your head to keep your neck and spine aligned.
- Take your arms down by your sides and keep them relaxed.
- Make sure you're in Neutral Spine – perform a few gentle pelvic tilts to find the correct position and then relax.

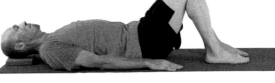

- Engage your abdominal muscles/pelvic floor muscles.
- Breathe in to your ribcage to prepare.
- Breathe out through your mouth while raising one leg into Table Top, so your knee is directly over your hip and your shin is parallel to the ceiling.
- Point your toes if it is comfortable to do so.

- Breathe in and, keeping your leg in this 90-degree angle and moving from the hip, lower your foot slowly and smoothly to the ground.

- Breathe out and return the leg, with control, to Table Top.
- Repeat for a total of up to 4 times either side.

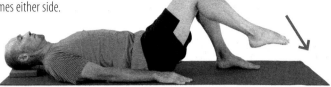

Note:
- Pay attention to your pelvis: make sure it's not moving around and that your back isn't arching as you lower your leg to the floor.
- Keep your abdominal muscles engaged and the rest of your body relaxed and chest open with your shoulders softly into your back.
- Concentrate on your breathing to help the exercise flow.

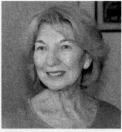

CASE STUDY

Janet Carr
Age: 74
Occupation: Customer service representative
Practised Pilates for: 15 years
Favourite exercise: the lying-down leg exercises

'First and foremost Pilates has helped improve my balance, which has given me greater confidence when walking. My core strength has improved immensely and I haven't suffered any sciatic pain which had troubled me for many years. The awareness of the need to stretch has helped me to stand tall – all 5ft 2in of me! Overall after a class I feel more energized and stimulated.'

DOUBLE KNEE FOLD

This is a progression from the Single Knee Fold (page 126). Make sure you can perform the Single Knee Fold and are comfortable with the process before moving on to this exercise.

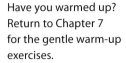
Have you warmed up? Return to Chapter 7 for the gentle warm-up exercises.

INTERMEDIATE/ADVANCED

Method

- Lie on your back.
- Place a block or small cushion under your head to keep your neck and spine aligned.
- Take your arms down by your sides and keep them relaxed.
- Bend your knees.
- Place your feet in line with your hips.
- Perform a few gentle pelvic tilts and come into Neutral Spine.
- Engage your abdominal muscles/pelvic floor muscles.
- Breathe in to your ribcage to prepare.
- Breathe out and raise one leg into Table Top.

- Breathe in and hold.
- Breathe out and raise your other leg into Table Top.

- Make sure both your knees are sitting above your hips.
- Point your toes as long as you are comfortable to do so.
- Breathe in to prepare.
- Breathe out and lower one foot to the floor, keeping the 90-degree angle of the leg.

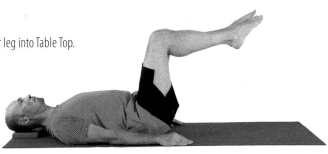

- Breathe in and return it to the start position.
- Breathe out and lower your other foot to the floor.

- Breathe in and return it to the start position.
- Continue alternating for up to a total of 6 repetitions.
- When you've completed the exercise, take one foot down to the mat at a time, taking care not to arch your back.

Note:
- Check that your abdominal muscles aren't doming as you perform the exercise and that your back isn't arching. Keep your abdominal muscles activated throughout.
- Make sure the knee isn't just bending more to tap the toe down – the movement should come from the hip joint hinging the leg down. Maintain the angle at the knee joint.
- If you find your back beginning to arch, don't take your foot down so low – stop halfway until you feel stronger.

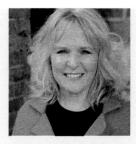

CASE STUDY
Valerie Dornbach
Age: 65
Occupation: Actor
Practised Pilates for: 10 years
Favourite exercise: Side Kick and Shoulder Bridge (pages 110 and 146)

'I run, so to do a Pilates class is better than a massage! I walk a lot too and can bend easily to pick up a ball for the dog. I am so much more flexible. When I had ITB problems, Pilates came to the rescue. When you are fit and well Pilates keeps you there, it recharges the batteries. It is the base from which my fitness takes root and grows. I stand up tall now and am so very aware if I start to slump and will correct it almost immmedietaly. It's really helped my posture when I run too.'

ARMS AND SHOULDERS SERIES

SHOULDER STABILITY

Benefits

The following simple and relaxing exercises will train your shoulders to stay in a neutral position – no tense shoulders rising up around your ears when you're out walking. You will also be stretching your *trapezius* (upper back) muscles and mobilizing your shoulder blades, ensuring your shoulders move more freely during everyday activities. If you perform these exercises with light hand weights (see Advanced) you will also be strengthening your arms too. Our upper body tends to be less strong than our lower body, and this imbalance can increase as we age. So it's important to keep using those muscles making it possible for us to continue to take part in the activities we enjoy or just simply carry our shopping bags or lift our grandchildren with ease.

ALL LEVELS

Method

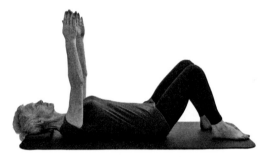

- Lie on your back.
- Bend your knees, feet in line with your hips.
- Come into Neutral Spine.
- Breathe naturally.
- Raise your arms straight up above your chest with palms facing inwards.

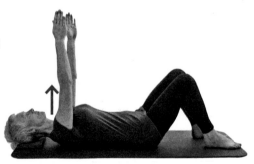

- Engage your abdominal muscles/pelvic floor muscles.
- Gently lift your shoulders off the floor as if you're trying to reach the ceiling with your fingertips

- Keeping your arms fully lengthened, shrug your shoulders gently back down to the floor.
- Repeat the movement slowly, up to 10 times in total.
- Return to the start position ready to go into the Arms and Shoulders exercise (page 131).

Note:

- Be aware of the rest of your body – when you lift your arms and shoulders, make sure the rest of the torso isn't going with you and that it stays stable.
- Try not to crash your shoulders back down on to the floor; keep the exercise flowing and controlled.
- Keep your neck and head stable.

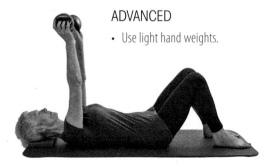

ADVANCED

- Use light hand weights.

ARMS AND SHOULDERS

Note: if you have shoulder problems, please modify by following the instructions towards the end of this exercise.

Method

- Lie on your back.
- Bend your knees, feet in line with your hips.
- Come into Neutral Spine.
- Raise your arms straight up above your chest with palms facing inwards.

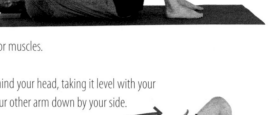

- Engage your abdominal muscles/ pelvic floor muscles.
- Breathe in to prepare.
- Breathe out and lengthen one arm back behind your head, taking it level with your ear (no further) and simultaneously take your other arm down by your side.
- Breathe in and hold the position.
- Breathe out and, keeping the movement smooth, swap your arms over.

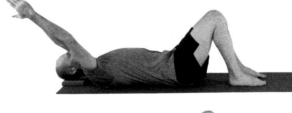

- Repeat for a total of up to 10 times.
- Return to the start position ready to go into Arms, Shoulders and Spinal Mobility (page 132).

Shoulder problems? Try this:

- If it's uncomfortable or painful to take your arm back level with your ear, just take it to a comfortable position which may be just a little way back – listen to your body and don't force it.

ADVANCED

- Use light hand weights.

Note:

- Keep your torso stable, remain in Neutral Spine and make sure you don't arch your back as you take your arm back.

- Try and straighten your arms, stretching the triceps (back of the arms) in the process, but keep your elbow slightly soft.

- Make sure your arm doesn't hug your head as you take it back – leave a space between your shoulder and your ear. Think about the alignment.

ARMS, SHOULDERS AND SPINAL MOBILITY

Method

- Lie on your back.
- Bend your knees, feet in line with your hips.
- Come into Neutral Spine.
- Raise your arms straight up above your chest with palms facing inwards.

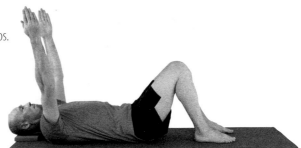

- Engage your abdominal muscles/ pelvic floor muscles.
- Breathe in to prepare.
- Breathe out and take both arms back behind your head no further than your ears.

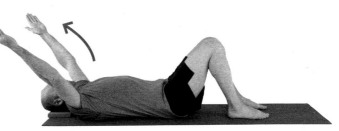

- Breathe in and hold the stretch but keep your torso in Neutral Spine.
- Breathe out and bring your arms back above your chest and then lower both down to your sides.
- Repeat up to 10 times.
- Return your arms to the centre, above your chest, ready to go into Arm Circles (page 134).

ADVANCED

- Use light hand weights, paying special attention to your alignment. Your back will want to arch against the weight of your arms even more now, so keep in Neutral Spine and down on the floor and your abdominal muscles engaged.

Note:

- Be aware of any spinal arching – your back will want to arch as you take both arms back. Imagine tucking your bottom rib into your trousers.
- Keep your abdominals engaged and your spine stable.
- If you find your back is beginning to arch and your ribs lift up, don't take your arms so far back.

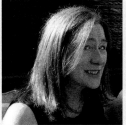

CASE STUDY

Sarah Macintyre
Age: 53
Occupation: Business development manager
Practised Pilates for: 2 years
Favourite exercise: Arm exercises with weights

'I started Pilates for general health reasons. I had heard about Pilates but wasn't sure what it was. I took advantage of a trial session and loved it. I do some recreational rowing which is very core strength based – the combination of that and Pilates complement each other.

I had a very bad frozen shoulder, with no movement at all at some points, so I had a steroid injection, which gave me movement again. But since doing Pilates I've not needed any more treatment. I now make more of an effort to think about my posture and stand taller. And I'm definitely more flexible, with fewer aches and pains and stiffness. I think Pilates exercises can be done at all ages, it really is for everyone.'

ARM CIRCLE

Benefits

Arm Circles improve both shoulder mobility and stabilization. This exercise will also challenge the steadiness of your torso, as it may want to move with your arms – it is a great exercise for training it to stay stable while we move our limbs, which is what we want it to do when we're walking or jogging. It will release tension around your neck and shoulders. You'll also find that, if you're a golfer or play tennis, your arm swing will improve as the shoulders become more flexible and mobile.

Note: if you have a shoulder problem, please keep these rotations small or omit the exercise.

Method

- Lie on your back in Neutral Spine.
- Bend your knees, feet in line with your hips.
- Breathe naturally.
- Raise your arms straight up above your chest with palms facing inwards.

- Engage your abdominal muscles/pelvic floor muscles.
- Begin rotating both arms from the shoulders, drawing a circle on the ceiling with your fingertips as long as your shoulders are comfortable.

- Rotate in one direction a few times, then rotate the other way.
- Come back to centre and stop circling.
- Breathe in to your ribcage.
- Breathe out through your mouth as you begin to make the circles bigger.
- Keep the lateral thoracic breathing going as you increase the range of movement, taking the arms behind your head and all the way round to your sides and then back up above your chest.

- Make a full circle on each breath.
- Complete up to 5 circles as long as your shoulders are comfortable, then change direction.

ADVANCED

- Use light hand weights. Make sure you stay in Neutral Spine and that the weights don't alter your exercise form or alignment.
- Increase the repetitions and range of movement but don't take the arms further back than your ears.

Note:
- Keep your abdominals engaged and your spine stable.
- If you find your back is beginning to arch and your ribs lift up, keep the rotations small.
- Keep the rest of the body relaxed and centred.

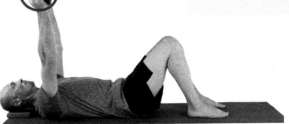

CASE STUDY

Hilary Bentley
Age: 66
Practised Pilates for: 3 years
Favourite exercises: Shoulder Bridge (page 146) for my back mobility, and arm exercises with weights to improve my arm strength.

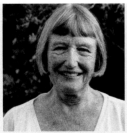

'I originally started Pilates to keep supple and improve my pelvic floor muscles. I walk and cycle, and Pilates gives me more energy and strength. It really helped strengthen the shoulder I broke a year ago too. Pilates also helps me maintain my back mobility and made me more aware of my posture, so I strive to lengthen and stand tall. Levels of energy have definitely gone up and I feel it has a calming effect too. I think it helps with total body awareness which helps me so much every day.'

DEAD BUG

Have you warmed up?
Return to Chapter 7
for the gentle warm-up
exercises.

Benefits

A relaxing but energizing exercise that lengthens nearly all the muscles in your body and helps to make you more aware of torso stability. This will transfer to all your activities, encouraging torso stability while your arms and legs move. Think back to the tree trunk on page 15 – the arms and legs are branches waving around and it's vital that you keep the trunk and roots stable. This exercise also strengthens your back, arms and leg muscles and can be made more challenging by using light hand and leg weights.

ALL LEVELS

Method

- Lie on your back.
- Place your arms down by your sides.
- Bend your knees, feet in line with your hips.
- Come into Neutral Spine.
- Engage your abdominal muscles/pelvic floor muscles.
- Take your right leg into Table Top.
- Raise your left arm above your chest with the palm of your hand facing inwards.

- Breathe in to prepare.
- Breathe out and lengthen your arm back behind your head, simultaneously extending your leg out in front of you, pointing your toes.

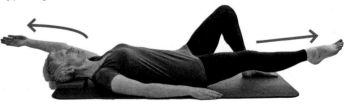

- Only take your arm back level with your ear, no further.
- Take your leg as low as you can but, if you feel your back begin to arch, raise your leg slightly higher.
- Breathe in, holding the lengthened position.
- Breathe out and slowly, with control, return the arm and leg back to the start position.
- Repeat up to 8 times in total and then change sides.

ADVANCED

- This exercise can be performed with light hand weights, but make sure when you take your arm back that it is stable.
- The same applies to the legs: you can use leg/ankle weights, although I would suggest starting with just hand weights to begin with. You are more likely to feel the back arch if you are wearing an ankle weight, so concentrate on keeping the pelvis stable and spine in neutral.
- Increase repetitions.

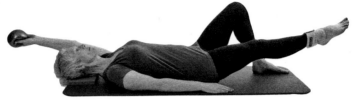

Note:
- Leave a space between your ear and arm when you lengthen it – don't hug your head.
- Try to stretch your triceps (back of the upper arms) as you lengthen your arm but keep your elbow soft.
- Concentrate on your breathing to help the exercise flow.
- Stay in Neutral Spine – be aware of any change in your alignment as you move your arms and legs.

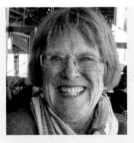

CASE STUDY

Caroline O'Connor
Age: 70
Practised Pilates for: 5 years
Favourite exercises: Difficult to say! Dead Bug and the social aspect!

'I'm sure Pilates has helped my tennis. I feel stronger and have more stamina than I used to have. My back is stronger – I used to have lower back pain and I rarely do now. I am much more aware of standing tall and maintaining good posture.

I love coming to class. The classes help physically and mentally, because it's good to spend time concentrating on certain exercises and movements. I regularly recommend Pilates to friends and family, particularly those with muscle pain or movement problems.'

THE HUNDRED (PREPARATION)

Benefits

The Hundred is a classic Pilates exercise that improves circulation and deep abdominal and lower back strength. It also enhances pelvic and shoulder stability, while challenging the leg and hip muscles. It's called The Hundred because it involves one hundred gentle beats of the arms. It's an all-over core strengthener that is a must for all of us. Weak abdominals just can't support your back, so this is a good place to start. It's also a good breathing exercise.

Before you perform the full exercise it's a good idea to practise the preparation. The Hundred can be an intense and challenging exercise and so it's important to get the process and alignment correct. Joseph Pilates described it as a 'warm-up exercise' – the breathing and pumping arms certainly gets the blood flowing, and was used to warm the body in preparation for the classic repertoire.

ALL LEVELS

Method

Part 1

- Lie on your back, knees bent and feet in line with the hips.
- Perform a few pelvic tilts and come into Neutral Spine.
- Engage your abdominal muscles/pelvic floor muscles.

- Breathe into your ribcage to prepare.
- Breathe out as you raise your head, curling up and lengthening through your neck to fix your gaze on your thighs.
- Lift and lengthen your arms a little way off the floor, palms down, level with your shoulders.

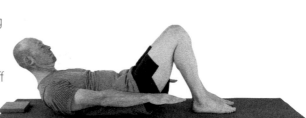

- Breathe in and hold the position.
- Breathe out and gently lower your head, neck and arms back down to the floor.

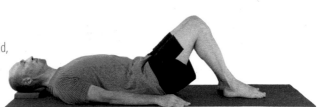

- Repeat the exercise a few more times and move on to Part 2 only when you feel comfortable with this first part, and your neck is not taking any tension.

Too challenging? Try this:
- If you're not comfortable with the neck flexion (lifting your head and looking towards your thighs
  – see page 140 for a note on this) then return to the Starter Pack and practise the Neck Curl-Ups
  supporting your head with your hand (page 70).

INTERMEDIATE/ADVANCED

Part 2

As long as you are not feeling any tension in your neck, are comfortable with neck flexion and you can
feel your abdominal muscles working, progress to this next stage. If you have a neck problem of any sort,
omit this part of this exercise.
- Lie on your back, knees bent and feet in line with the hips.
- Perform a few pelvic tilts and come into Neutral Spine.
- Engage your abdominal muscles/pelvic floor muscles.
- Breathe in to prepare.
- Breathe out as you raise your head,
  curling up and lengthening through
  your neck to fix your gaze on your thighs.
- Breathe in and raise your arms up to
  shoulder level, palms down.

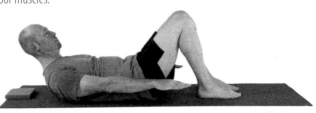

- Breathe out and, keeping your
  head and neck in the same
  position, take your arms back
  behind you (no further than your
  ears) and lengthen.
- Breathe in holding the position.
  Look down towards your thighs
  rather than up to the ceiling.

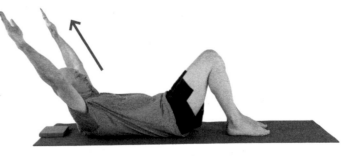

- Breathe out, float the arms back
  towards the hips and gently lower
  your head, neck and arms back
  down to the floor.

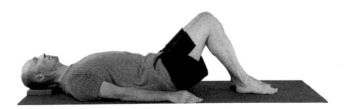

- Rock your head gently from side to side to release any tension.
- Repeat 2 times, as long as you are using your abdominal muscles and not
  straining your neck.

▶ ▶

Note:
- If you feel a lot of tension in your neck, do not take your arms so far back; they can stay just above your chest or you can just release down to the mat and complete the first part of this exercise.
- Engaging your abdominal muscles before you breathe in and move will help.
- Imagine you have an apple or tennis ball under your chin and you are trying to hold it there as you perform the exercise and look towards your thighs.

- Come into a Full Body Stretch before performing The Hundred.

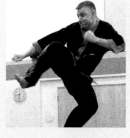

CASE STUDY

Graham Parks
Age: 50
Occupation: Tae Kwon Do instructor
Practised Pilates for: 3 years
Favourite exercise: The Hundred

'I started Pilates because the non-weight bearing element of it complimented my Tae Kwon Do practice and the fact that as I've grown older my joints have become stiffer. My core strength has improved – it's always been quite good but I've really noticed a difference. My flexibility and muscular control has improved too. In 2015 I ruptured my Anterior Cruciate Ligament in an accident and Pilates has been a major part of my rehabilitation process. The exercises have complimented the ones my physio recommended – stability of the knee, using muscles to reconnect, that sort of thing. I also love the "mental" side of Pilates, the mindfulness aspect – it gives me space.'

THE HUNDRED

INTERMEDIATE

Method

- Lie on your back, knees bent, feet in line with the hips.
- Perform a few pelvic tilts and come into Neutral Spine or imprint your spine on to the mat.
- Engage your abdominal muscles/pelvic floor muscles.
- Raise one leg at a time into Table Top.

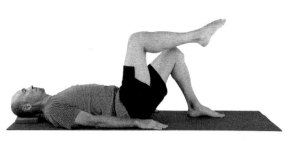

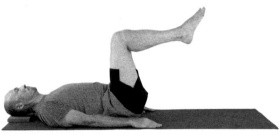

- Breathe in to prepare.
- Breathe out as you raise your head, curling up and lengthening through your neck to fix your gaze on your thighs.
- Raise your arms up to the same height as your shoulders, palms down.

- Breathe in for 5 beats as you gently pulse your arms, moving from your shoulders.
- Breathe out for 5 beats.
- Repeat until you have completed 100 gentle pulses with your arms.

Note:
- If you feel tension in your neck or have a neck problem, put your head down.
- Keep those abdominal muscles/pelvic floor muscles engaged throughout.
- Imagine you have something delicate under your hands as you pulse; keep the movement small.
- Concentrate on your breathing to help the exercise flow.

Too challenging? Try this:
- If you find 100 beats too many to start with, then aim for 30, 40 or 50 and build up.
- Alternatively, perform the exercise without raising your head or arms. Engage the abdominal muscles and hold the legs stable in Table Top, making sure your back doesn't arch – you'll still be working the TVA.

- Focus on your lateral thoracic breathing.
- When you feel strong enough, try raising your head, neck and arms for a short while.

SINGLE LEG STRETCH

BEGINNER/INTERMEDIATE

Benefits

This exercise will strengthen your core muscles, increase flexibility and challenge your coordination. It stretches the hamstrings (back of thighs), abdominal muscles, glutes, neck and hip flexors. The hip flexors help raise the leg – think how often they have to do that when you're walking, and how hard they need to work! If you sit at a desk all day, your hip flexors (as well as your hamstrings and glutes) can become tight, so it's important to strengthen and lengthen them as they are often neglected and then, as we age, we begin to suffer.

Method

- Lie on your back.
- Bend your knees, feet in line with your hips.
- Perform a few pelvic tilts to find your Neutral Spine.
- Engage your abdominal muscles/ pelvic floor muscles.
- Raise first one leg and then the other leg into Table Top.

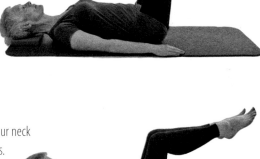

- Raise your head, lengthening through your neck so that you're looking towards your knees.

- Place your hands lightly either side of one thigh or calf.
- Extend the other leg out in front of you, hovering above the floor, pointing your toes.

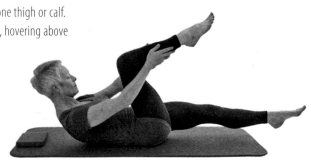

- Breathe in to prepare.
- Breathe out and swap the legs over, moving your hands from leg to leg as you do so and keeping your neck flexed as you look towards your knees.

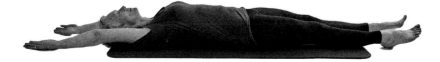

- Continue slowly in a controlled manner, using lateral thoracic breathing, or breathing naturally if you find it easier. Avoid holding your breath.
- Complete up to 16 repetitions – although once again, work up to this amount of repetitions if it's too much for now, it won't take you long. Then take your head and neck down to the floor before lowering first one leg and then the other. Come into a Full Body Stretch.

Note:

- Keep your abdominal muscles engaged and try to keep the torso stable – avoid bobbing from side to side, keep your eye focus central.
- Try and keep the rest of the body relaxed – soften your shoulders away from your ears.

- Don't hold your breath – if you find the lateral thoracic breathing challenging, try short out breaths every time your leg returns.

Too challenging? Try this:
- Keep your head and neck down on the mat and just lengthen the legs.
- If you find your back arching, then move your lower leg higher when you extend it out in front of you.

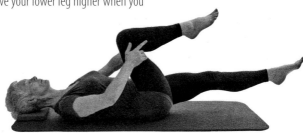

DOUBLE LEG STRETCH

ADVANCED

Note: *if you have neck problems, please take care – see modifications towards end of exercise.*

Benefits

This is a more challenging exercise than Single Leg Stretch (page 142). It requires good abdominal strength and control to maintain alignment. Please only attempt this exercise if you feel strong enough. Like Single Leg Stretch this exercise will strengthen your core muscles, increase flexibility and challenge your coordination. It stretches the hamstrings, abdominal muscles, glutes, neck and hip flexors. When your hip flexors are lengthened, any tightness you might feel in your hamstrings, ITB or quads should start to release.
In addition, this is a good shoulder mobilizer and will release any tension.

Method

- Lie on your back, knees bent and feet in line with the hips.
- Come into Neutral Spine.
- Engage your abdominal muscles/pelvic floor muscles.
- Raise first one leg and then your other leg into Table Top.

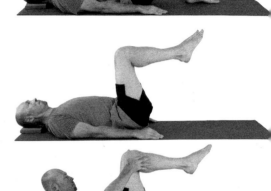

- Raise your head, lengthening through your neck so that you're looking towards your knees.
- Place your hands lightly around either side of both your knees.

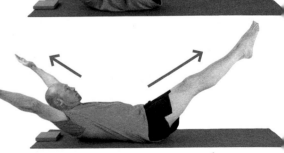

- Breathe in to your ribcage to prepare.
- Breathe out, lengthening your arms behind you as far as your ears, and simultaneously lengthening your legs out at an angle of about 45 degrees to the floor.
- Squeeze your inner thighs together.

- Breathe in and return to the start position, keeping your head and neck in the flexed position.

- Breathe out and repeat the movement, lengthening your arms behind and legs out in front.

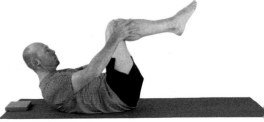

- Repeat up to 10 times and then bring your arms down by your sides. Lower your head, and then take one leg at a time down to the floor. Come into a Full Body Stretch.

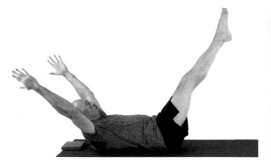

Note:
- Make sure your back does not arch; keep your abdominals engaged throughout.
- If your back is arching, keep your legs a little higher until you are stronger.
- Keep your eyes on your knees; don't let your neck and head drop back.

Too challenging? Neck tension? Try this:
- Take your arms only halfway back and keep your legs higher.

- If your neck is feeling tense, take your head down to the floor.
- Only extend the legs, omit the arm movement. Or just perform the Single Leg Stretch (page 142).

Want even more of a challenge? Try this:
- Increase repetitions.
- Slow the exercise right down.
- Circle your arms around to the sides of your body to bring them back to the starting position, simultaneously bring your knees back to your torso.

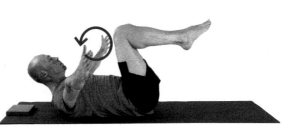

SHOULDER BRIDGE

Benefits

The Shoulder Bridge is another brilliant and popular exercise that teaches torso stability, lengthens the spine and has the added benefit of strengthening and activating lazy buttock muscles. When walking, especially long distance and power walking or jogging, our glutes often let us down, either because they're not firing properly or are weak. This can cause all sorts of problems and is often the cause of lumbar and pelvic instability (as discussed in Chapter 5). If you want to power up those hills, strengthen those glutes! The Shoulder Bridge also encourages spinal alignment, mobility, and stretches the back muscles and quads (front of thighs) while strengthening the hamstrings (back of thighs) and core muscles. It opens up the hips and lengthens the hip flexors.

It's a great exercise to do after a long walk, sporting session, or if you've been gardening and bending over a lot. It will help to lengthen and relax a tight, achy back and hamstrings. It undoes all those knotty tension spots in your back. Stick to the basic beginner exercise rather than the progressions if you're just using it as a good all round stretch and relax.

In addition, if you have a groin or hamstring injury, Shoulder Bridge, because of its torso-stabilizing movement, is excellent as a rehabilitation exercise.

ALL LEVELS

Method

- Lie on your back, knees bent, feet in line with the hips.
- Place a block or cushion under your head if you need it to keep your neck and spine aligned.
- Relax your arms down by your sides.

- Perform a few pelvic tilts to find your Neutral Spine.
- Activate your glutes (by squeezing) and engage your abdominal muscles/pelvic floor muscles.
- Breathe in to your ribcage to prepare.
- Breathe out as you slowly curl from the base of your spine, off the floor, one vertebrae at a time towards the ceiling.

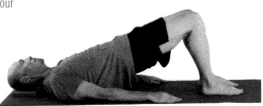

- Breathe in at the top.
- Breathe out as you gently and slowly lower your spine back down to the floor, one vertebrae at a time.
- Repeat up to 8 times and then come into a Full Body Stretch.

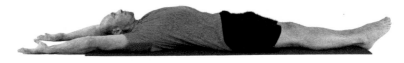

Note:

- Make sure your hips don't come higher than your knees when your spine is lifted off the floor – check that you have a straight line from knees to shoulders.

- Keep the weight evenly distributed between your feet.
- Be aware of any wobble – try to keep your torso steady throughout.

- Keep those abdominal and glute muscles engaged throughout.
- Concentrate on your breathing to help the exercise flow.

INTERMEDIATE

This progression of Shoulder Bridge challenges your coordination as well as improving shoulder mobility. If you choose to use light hand weights, you will also be working your arms and increasing the challenge of keeping your torso stable.

- Lie on your back, knees bent, feet in line with the hips.
- Relax your arms down by your sides, with weights if you are using them.
- Perform a few pelvic tilts and come into Neutral Spine.
- Engage your glutes and abdominal muscles/pelvic floor muscles.
- Breathe in to your ribcage to prepare.
- Breathe out as you lift both your arms, extending them backwards. At the same time slowly curl from the base of your spine, off the floor, one vertebrae at a time towards the ceiling.

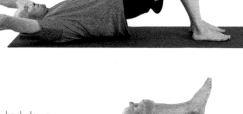

- Breathe in at the top.
- Breathe out as you simultaneously take your arms slowly back down to the mat while gently lowering your spine down to the floor.
- Repeat up to 10 times. When you have completed the repetitions and have come back down to the floor, bring both your knees into your chest and give them a hug.

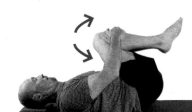

- Rotate your knees first one way and then the other, which has the effect of massaging your lower back, before coming into a Full Body Stretch.

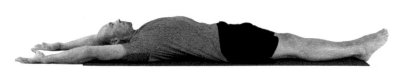

Want more of a challenge? Try this:

This progression of Shoulder Bridge has the added benefit of an abdominal curl included at the end. The coordination of this exercise is more challenging than the previous versions, but really good for us. So take the exercise slowly and try to keep the movements flowing.

- Lie on your back, knees bent, feet in line with the hips.
- Relax your arms down by your sides, with weights if you are using them.
- Perform a few pelvic tilts and come into Neutral Spine.
- Engage your glutes and abdominal muscles/pelvic floor muscles.
- Breathe in to your ribcage to prepare.
- Breathe out as you lift both your arms, extending them backwards. At the same time slowly curl from the base of your spine, off the floor, one vertebrae at a time towards the ceiling.

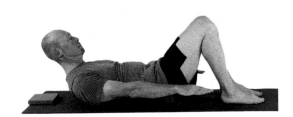

- Breathe in at the top.
- Breathe out as you simultaneously take your arms slowly back towards the mat and return your spine to the floor. When your glutes reach the mat, raise your head and neck and look towards your knees or thighs.

- Breathe in as you hold the position.
- Breathe out as your take your head back down to the floor and start to curl back up into Shoulder Bridge.

ADVANCED

This advanced version of Shoulder Bridge works those glute muscles even harder by increasing the pelvic stability challenge. It also targets all the core muscles.

- Lie on your back, knees bent, feet in line with the hips.
- Relax your arms down by your sides with weights if you are using them.
- Perform a few pelvic tilts to come into Neutral Spine.
- Engage your glutes and abdominal muscles/pelvic floor muscles.
- Breathe in to your ribcage to prepare.
- Slowly curl from the base of your spine, off the floor, one vertebrae at a time towards the ceiling.

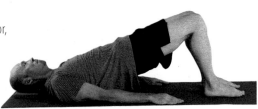

- Breathe naturally.
- In the raised Shoulder Bridge position, lift one foot off the floor.
- Bend the knee towards your chest.

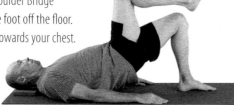

Note:

- Keep your pelvis stable and hips level — if you notice that you are tilting to one side, lift the glute back up into the correct position.
- Be aware of torso stability and what the rest of your body is doing. Correct any wobbling that might be going on.
- Keep abdominal muscles and glutes engaged throughout.
- Sometimes this exercise can cause cramping in the hamstrings particularly if you are prone to cramp. This often happens if the glutes aren't being activated enough or are weak — the hamstrings take over. So make sure you are squeezing those buttock muscles.

- Straighten the leg towards the ceiling, pointing your toes.

- Breathe in, holding that position.
- Breathe out and lower your raised leg to the same height as the bent knee.

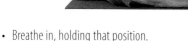

- Breathe in and lift your raised leg up to the ceiling, again keeping your hips stable.
- Repeat 4 times.
- Bend your knee back towards your chest and lower your foot to the ground and then gently curl your spine back down to the floor.

- Repeat on the other side 4 times. Bring both your knees into your chest and hug them. Rotate first one way and then the other, massaging your lower back in the process. Come into a Full Body Stretch.

SINGLE LEG BRIDGE

Benefits

This is another development of the fantastic Shoulder Bridge but a more advanced exercise, with the added challenge of performing the exercise one side at a time. As well as all the same benefits of the full Shoulder Bridge, the Single Leg Bridge challenges stability and control of the pelvis even more and can show up any imbalances in the glutes and hip area. For example, you might find that one side feels stronger than the other as you perform the exercise, an indication that glute strength is unequal. Or you might find that on one side the hip flexors feel less comfortable.

ADVANCED

Method

- Lie on your back, knees bent, feet in line with the hips.
- Relax your arms down by your sides.
- Come into Neutral Spine.
- Engage your abdominal muscles/pelvic floor muscles and glutes.
- Breathe in to prepare.
- Breathe out and gently peel your spine off the mat and into Shoulder Bridge (page 146).

Note:

- Make sure you keep your hips level.
- Keep your abdominal muscles and glutes engaged throughout.
- Concentrate on keeping the rest of the body relaxed and use your breathing to help the exercise flow.

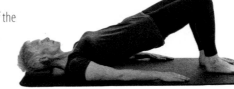

- Breathe in at the top.
- Breathe out and take one foot off the floor, lengthening the leg to the ceiling and pointing your toes.

- Breathe in and lower your spine slowly and with control back down to the floor.

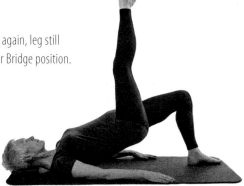

- Breathe out and peel your spine off the floor again, leg still raised, until you come back into the Shoulder Bridge position.
- Repeat up to 6 times and then change legs.

- Bring both knees into your chest and give them a hug, rotating first one way and then the other, which has the effect of massaging your lower back. Then come into a Full Body Stretch.

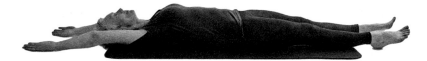

Too challenging? Try this:
- Return to the Shoulder Bridge (page 146) and familiarize yourself with that exercise again. When you feel stronger, come back and try this exercise again.

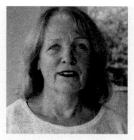

CASE STUDY

Denise Head
Age: 64
Practised Pilates for: 8 years
Favourite exercise: The warm-up routine gives a good overall stretch and activates muscles that I may not otherwise use, especially in the neck, back, hips and feet.

'I started Pilates to improve overall muscle tone, balance and core strength. Mentally, Pilates is such a great way to spend some 'me' time – exercising while relaxing to some gentle background mood music and focusing on my own wellbeing. Physically, Pilates has helped improve my balance, range of joint movement, core muscle strength and flexibility. These are all really important to maintain if we want to continue to enjoy a busy and active lifestyle. Specifically though, Pilates has helped to relieve tight muscles in my back, neck and hips. I often do the simple stretching exercises – full body stretch, leg lengthening from the hip and neck exercises – in bed, if discomfort in these areas keep me awake. Also, Pilates is easy to do any place, any time, even on holiday, as most of the exercises do not require any special equipment.'

HIP CIRCLE

Benefits

This exercise improves hip mobility, strengthens the hip flexors, the adductor (inside thigh) muscles, the abductor (outside thigh) muscles and the core muscles. While circling the leg (or knee if you're a beginner) you'll be focused on hip and pelvis stability, which can be quite challenging but brings about an awareness of how easy it is for the pelvis to be unstable when walking, jogging or playing sport. This is also a good exercise for stretching those tight hamstrings (back of thighs) after a long walk or hike.

BEGINNER

Method

- Lie on your back, knees bent, feet in line with the hips.
- Place a block or cushion under your head to keep your neck and spine aligned if you need it.
- Relax your arms down by your sides.
- Come into Neutral Spine.
- Engage your abdominal muscles/pelvic floor muscles.
- Raise your right leg into Table Top and rest your right hand or fingers lightly on your knee.

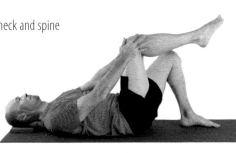

- Breathe in to prepare.
- Breathe out and circle your knee in towards your body guiding it with your hand and then out away from the body.

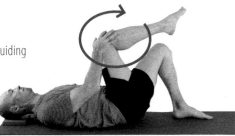

- Breathe in and keep circling.
- Continue to circle for 5 times in total using your breathing and keeping the movement smooth and continuous.
- Reverse the movement and then repeat on the other side.

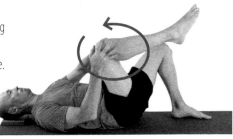

- Make sure your hip does not come off the floor as you rotate.
- Be aware of your pelvic stability.
- Keep the movement flowing and smooth.
- If you find the pelvis moves around, keep the circles small to start with.
- Keep your abdominal muscles engaged and be aware of what the bent knee is doing. Is it flailing around and joining in? If so, stabilize!

BEGINNER/INTERMEDIATE with Dyna-Band™ or yoga strap
Method
- Lie on your back, knees bent, feet in line with the hips.
- Hook the band around the sole of one foot, extend the leg to the ceiling while holding the ends of the band in the hand on the same side.
- Take your other arm out to the side to stabilize your torso.

- Engage your abdominal muscles/pelvic floor muscles and maintain Neutral Spine.
- Breathe in to your ribcage to prepare.
- Breathe out and gently and slowly guide your leg around in a circle keeping the pelvis stable.

- Start off small and then if you feel confident and your pelvis remains stable make the circle larger, sweeping your leg around to the side and then across your body guiding it with your Dyna-band. Aim for 4 rotations in total as long as you feel comfortable to do so.
- Reverse and then repeat on the other side.

Note:
- Place your other hand on your hip so that you can feel any movement in the pelvis.

- Make sure your hip does not come off the floor as you rotate.
- The larger the circle, the more challenging it will be, so be aware of your pelvic stability.
- Keep the movement flowing and smooth.
- If you find the pelvis moves around, keep the circles small to start with.
- Keep your abdominal muscles engaged and be aware of what the bent knee is doing. Is it flailing around and joining in? If so, stabilize!

ADVANCED

Method

- Lie on your back, knees bent, feet in line with the hips.
- Relax your arms down by your sides.
- Come into Neutral Spine.
- Engage your abdominal muscles/pelvic floor muscles.
- Raise one leg and lengthen it to the ceiling, pointing your toes.

- Breathe in to your ribcage to prepare.
- Breathe out and, moving from the hip, draw small circles on the ceiling with your toes.
- Breathe in again, still circling the leg.
- Breathe out and reverse the movement, still keeping the circles small.

- Breathe in as you bring the leg back to centre.
- Breathe out and sweep the leg around to the side of your body, extend down to the front and across your torso, making a big, wide circular movement.

- Repeat using your lateral thoracic breathing and moving on your out breath for up to 4 rotations each way.
- Change legs and repeat.

- Make sure your hip does not come off the floor as you rotate.
- The larger the circle the more challenging it will be, so be aware of your pelvic stability.
- Keep the movement flowing and smooth.
- If you find the pelvis moves around, keep the circles small to start with.
- Keep your abdominal muscles engaged and be aware of what the bent knee is doing. Is it flailing around and joining in? If so, stabilize!

Note:
- Place your hands on your hips so that you can feel any movement in the pelvis.

Want more of a challenge? Try this:
- Increase repetitions.
- Draw larger circles, but make sure the pelvis isn't joining in and that your abdominal muscles stay engaged.

REVERSE LEG PULL/PLANK

Benefits

This challenging exercise will improve your general posture and strengthen your core, lower back, spine, hips, arms, shoulders and glutes. It opens out the chest, stretching the pectoral muscles. These can become tight during long hikes or if you've been gardening and bending over a lot, or if you spend your day hunched over a computer. It is also a wonderful exercise for stretching hip flexors, which can get very tired from all the repetitive leg lifting while walking or if you've been jogging. Your deltoid (upper arm) muscles will be strengthened as well. It also promotes stabilization in the shoulders and challenges spinal and pelvic stability.

> Have you warmed up? Return to Chapter 7 for the gentle warm-up exercises.

Note: if you have wrist, shoulder or neck problems, place your hands on a small cushion or omit this exercise.

INTERMEDIATE

Method

- Sit up tall on your **sit bones** with your knees bent in front of you and feet flat on the floor.
- Place your hands behind your buttocks with your fingers facing sideways.

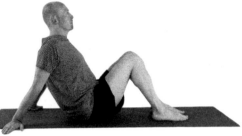

- Engage your abdominal muscles/pelvic floor muscles.
- Breathe in to prepare.
- Breathe out and lift your torso off the ground into a box position.
- Keep your head facing forwards, chin towards your chest.

- Breathe in and hold the position.
- Breathe out and lengthen first one leg and then the other leg out in front of you.

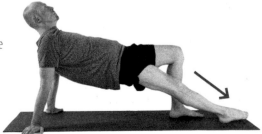

- Use your lateral thoracic breathing and hold for 3 breaths.
- Breathe in again.

- Breathe out and slowly lower yourself back down to the floor with your legs still extended.

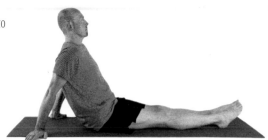

- Repeat up to 4 times and then come into a Full Body Stretch.

Note:
- For some, the hand position can be uncomfortable. Change direction, pointing your fingers away from your body if you find that to be more comfortable.

Too challenging? Try this:
- Perform fewer repetitions and hold for fewer breaths at the top.
- Complete the exercise by just lifting into the start position, with bent knees/box shape only. Repeat several times.

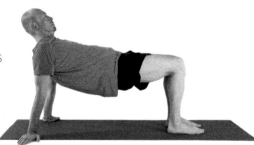

- Or just extend one leg at a time, returning to the bent knee position.

- Keep the hips and chest open and your torso stable.
- Concentrate on your breathing to help the exercise flow.

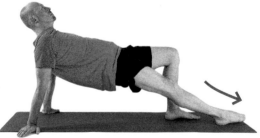

Note:
- As you become more confident with this progression, start to use the lateral thoracic breathing: breathe in when lifting the leg, breathe out when lowering it.

- Increase repetitions if you feel confident but keep your torso stable and chest open.
- Maintain a straight line from shoulders to toes; don't let your body sag.

ADVANCED

- Sit up tall on your 'sit bones' with your knees bent in front of you and feet flat on the floor.
- Place your hands behind your buttocks with your fingers facing sideways.

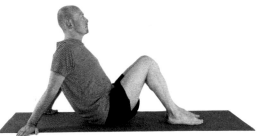

- Engage your abdominal muscles/pelvic floor muscles.
- Breathe in to your ribcage to prepare.
- Breathe out and lift your torso off the ground into a box position.
- Keep your head facing forwards, chin towards your chest.

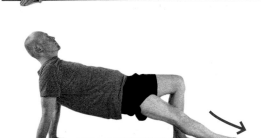

- Breathe in and hold the position.
- Breathe out and lengthen first one leg and then the other leg out in front of you.

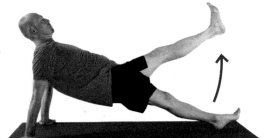

- Breathing naturally and from this extended leg position, quickly lift one leg up towards the ceiling, flexing your foot.

- Return it to the start position, pointing your toes.
- Repeat on the other side.
- Repeat up to 6 times in total or just attempt one or two to start with and then build up the repetitions. Bring your torso gently down to the floor and into Full Body Stretch.

SCISSORS

Benefits

This exercise will give your hamstrings (the muscles at the back of your thighs) a really good stretch. Sometimes these can be really tight if you sit a lot or have been walking up hills and your glutes aren't working hard enough! It will also mobilize your hips while strengthening your core muscles, encouraging the torso to remain stable as you dynamically and rhythmically move your legs, all the while challenging your coordination, building stamina and stretching your upper back and improving your posture.

Note: *if your hamstrings are very tight, modify as per the instructions towards the end of this exercise (however, if they are tight, they probably need a good stretch!).*

ALL LEVELS

Method

- Lie on your back.
- Bend both knees, feet in line with the hips.
- Come into Neutral Spine and make sure your body is relaxed with your arms down by your sides.
- Engage your abdominal muscles/pelvic floor muscles.
- Raise one leg and lengthen it to the ceiling, pointing your toes.
- Extend the other leg along the floor, pointing your toes.

- Curl your head and neck up and look towards your raised knee.
- Wrap your hands lightly around the sides of your calf or thigh.

- Breathe in to prepare.
- Breathe out and dynamically swap the legs over in a scissor action.
- Continue to scissor the legs, catching each calf or thigh in your hands as it elevates, with the legs crossing over in mid-air as you breathe in.

- Keep your lower leg hovering above the floor – putting it down on the floor is cheating!
- Repeat up to 16 scissor actions, as long as you are comfortable to do so.
- Finish by lowering your head to the floor and bringing both knees into your chest. Then take one leg at a time down to the floor before coming into Full Body Stretch.

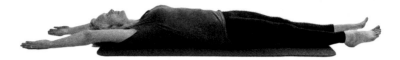

Note:

- Keep the pelvis stable and spine in neutral while you move your legs.
- If you find your pelvis is moving, slow the exercise down so that you can concentrate on the all-important stability.

- Your hands should be lightly touching each leg. Don't pull the leg – your abdominal muscles should be doing the work and engaged throughout.

Too challenging? Try this:

- If your hamstrings are very tight, bend your knees towards your chest a little.

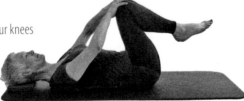

Neck feeling tense? Try this:

- If you find you are tensing your neck muscles and it's uncomfortable, put your head down and keep your arms by your sides. You can just move the legs and aim to improve the flexibility of the hamstrings while working on strengthening your core muscles.
- Keep in Neutral Spine, abdominals engaged throughout. Don't let your back arch – if it does, don't take your legs right down to the floor, let them hover halfway.

Want more of a challenge? Try this:

- Increase repetitions.
- Add a beat to the lower leg for the count of 2, but make sure the pelvis remains stable.

ROLLING LIKE A BALL

Benefits

This exercise mobilizes the lumbar spine (page 30), an area of the back that can become quite tight. It also massages and opens up all the back muscles, which can reduce any tension, and stretches the glutes (buttock muscles). In addition, this exercise improves abdominal strength and coordination. There is also the opportunity to challenge your balance as you progress to the advanced version of this exercise. You might have practised this exercise as a child, either on a trampoline or your own bed, or maybe you still do it now with your grandchildren! It has a wonderful freeing feeling to it.

Note: if you have serious back problems or bone density problems, please omit this exercise.

BEGINNER/INTERMEDIATE

Method

- Sit up tall on your 'sit bones'. Make sure you're using a mat because you will need the padding for your spine. Move yourself to the front edge so that you have space behind you to roll back. Please make sure you have moved any furniture out of the way because this is a dynamic exercise and it's quite easy to go off course when you first try it.
- Bend your knees, with feet flat on the floor.
- Rest your hands lightly on your shins and tuck your chin towards your chest.

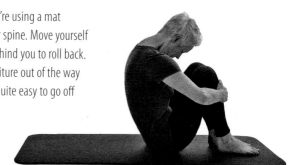

- Breathe in to prepare. Breathe out to stabilize and engage your abdominal muscles/pelvic floor muscles.
- Breathe in and roll yourself backwards like a ball, rolling no further than your shoulder blades.

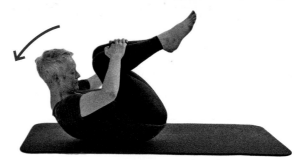

- Breathe out, deepen the abdominal connection and roll straight back up again and balance on your sit bones momentarily.

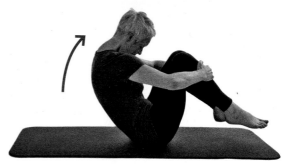

- Repeat up to 10 times as long as you are comfortable to do so, and then come into Full Body Stretch.

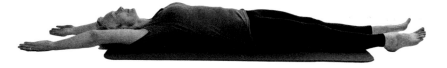

Note:

- Make sure you keep your chin tucked in to your chest and that you don't roll back on to your neck or head.
- Keep the breathing going and make sure your abdominal muscles are engaged throughout.
- Maintain your 'ball' shape throughout: make sure you don't kick your legs in the air or lose your eye focus. Look in towards your abdomen at all times.
- Try not to use your arms to pull yourself back up each time.

ADVANCED

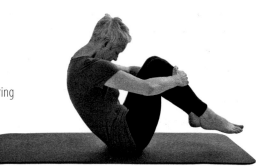

- Increase repetitions.
- Perform the exercise slowly with less momentum, which will require more abdominal control.
- Challenge your balance by keeping your feet hovering above the floor when you return to the sitting position – stop the wobble by engaging those abdominal muscles.

- Hold for longer at the top with your feet off the floor.

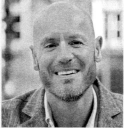

CASE STUDY

Matthew Bennet
Age: 48
Occupation: Managing Director
Practised Pilates for: 2 years
Favourite exercise: Leg Pull/Plank (page 88)

'I started Pilates because of my lower back pain and poor posture. I've seen a big improvement in my cycling stamina and core strength and I no longer get lower back pain when I swim. My back is completely pain free! And I'm taller – I now think to check my posture. It used to be difficult to stand for long periods, but no longer. I feel more energized and flexible, and able to lift and carry items more easily because of my stronger back. More than anything, it has reignited my passion for exercise in all forms, after a 5-year hiatus I'm now running again too.'

ROLL BACK

Have you warmed up?
Return to Chapter 7
for the gentle warm-up
exercises.

Benefits

This exercise strengthens the abdominal and hip muscles. It's also a good exercise to start with if you find the Roll Up with Spinal Stretch (page 164) too challenging. Avoid this exercise if you have disc-related back issues.

ALL LEVELS

Method

- Sit up tall on your 'sit bones' and bend your knees, feet flat on the floor.
- Place your hands lightly around the sides of both thighs.

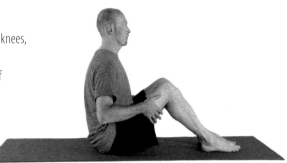

- Engage your abdominal muscles/pelvic floor muscles.
- Breathe in to prepare.
- Breathe out and slowly begin to round your back into a 'C' shape, scooping out your abdominal muscles. Keep your shoulders soft, away from your ears.

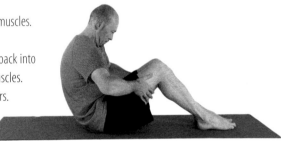

- Start to lower your lumbar spine, vertebrae by vertebrae, down towards the floor.
- Stop when you get to the point where you feel you might just drop back if you go any further. Keep your feet heavy: notice if your feet start to lift up off the floor.

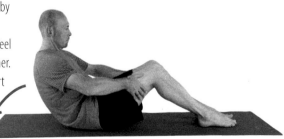

Note:

- Imagine sending your ribs down towards your hips as you scoop out your abdominal muscles.

- Keep your abdominal muscles engaged and when you return to the sitting position, lengthen through your spine into a fully upright position.

- Breathe in and hold the lowered position.
- Breathe out and slowly start to return to sitting position.
- Repeat up to 8 times and then come into a Full Body Stretch.

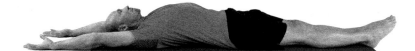

Not challenging enough? Try this:
- Increase the repetitions.
- Roll back with the aim of getting your spine closer to the floor.
- Flex your feet as you perform the exercise for an added calf stretch.

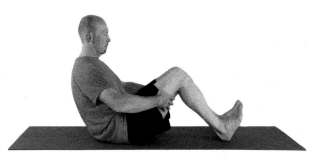

- Progress to Roll Up with Spinal Stretch (page 164).

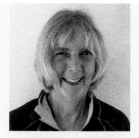

CASE STUDY

Sarah Gregory
Age: 63
Practised Pilates for: 6 years
Favourite exercise: Shoulder Bridge (page 146)

'I am much more flexible when I play tennis, I'm able to bend and stretch to reach the ball. And since doing Pilates I sleep better. Before, I was very stiff in my back and at night in bed I used to get fixed in a position unable to move without waking up and consciously moving very tentatively – this happens now only very rarely. When I am out walking I have a voice in my head that says "shoulders up, back and down into your back pockets" which helps my posture. My body feels much more flexible so I am not straining against it. I had a frozen shoulder which through Pilates is now completely better. I think everyone should do Pilates and they should teach it in schools so from a young age you begin to stretch and look after your body.'

ROLL UP WITH SPINAL STRETCH

Benefits

This exercise targets and strengthens the abdominal muscles and improves spinal and hamstring flexibility, which will increase your walking or jogging power. This exercise can be a challenge for some, so take your time and if you find that you can't quite get yourself off the floor into the Roll Up without momentum, take time to strengthen those abdominal muscles with other exercises and then return to this one when you feel confident.

INTERMEDIATE/ADVANCED

Method

- Lie on your back, legs extended.
- Take your arms above your head and rest them on the floor like in Full Body Stretch.

- Engage your abdominal muscles/pelvic floor muscles.
- Breathe in to prepare and raise your straight arms up above your chest.

- Breathe out and start to curl your head, neck and torso up off the floor until you reach a tall sitting position.

- Breathe in at the top.
- Breathe out and lengthen yourself forwards, stretching your arms towards your feet into a spinal stretch.

- Breathe in as you hold the stretch.
- Breathe out and lift your arms up, sitting upright, and then gently roll yourself back down, with control, to the lying position.

Note:

- Keep the movement slow and controlled – which is the hardest part. Use your breathing to help the exercise flow and keep lengthening through your spine as you engage those abdominal muscles.
- Don't let your legs lift up off the floor.
- Make sure you return to the lying position in a slow, controlled manner; try not to flop back down to the floor with relief!

Too challenging? Try this:

- If your abdominal muscles aren't quite strong enough and you find it hard to get yourself off the floor without adding momentum, try rolling up a small towel and placing it underneath your lower back – sometimes this works, especially if you have a lordotic lower back (page 30).

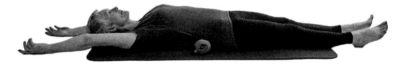

- Try performing the exercise with your knees bent.

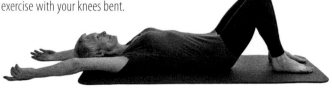

- Try the Roll Up with Dyna-Band™ which you may find easier to begin with (page 166).

ROLL UP WITH DYNA-BAND™

BEGINNER

Method

- Sit up tall on your 'sit bones' and bend your knees.
- Take your Dyna-Band™, hook it around the soles of your feet and extend your legs out in front of you. Toes pointing to the ceiling, heels planted on the floor.
- Hold on tight to the ends of the Dyna-Band™.

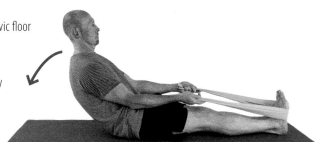

- Engage your abdominal muscles/pelvic floor muscles.
- Breathe in to prepare.
- Breathe out and lower yourself gently down to the floor, scooping out your abdominal muscles as you do so.

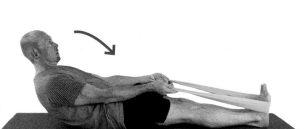

- Breathe in when you reach the floor.
- Breathe out and use the Dyna-Band™ to gently roll yourself up off the mat, slowly and with control, but make sure you aren't using your arms too much – those abdominal muscles need to work!

- Repeat up to 10 times as long as you are comfortable to do so.

Note:

- Keep your shoulders stabilized; try not to let them rise up around your ears when you are rolling yourself up to the sitting position.
- Engage your abdominal muscles throughout.
- Concentrate on your breathing to help the exercise flow.

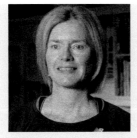

CASE STUDY

Sally Harvey
Age: 49
Occupation: Personal Assistant
Practised Pilates for: 4 years
Favourite exercise: Roll Down (page 51)

'I started Pilates because of my chronic and sometimes acute back pain. I can now do a lot more on a daily basis because I'm not going to be in pain afterwards. Pilates has given me freedom to play sport and run a half-marathon. It also gives me a "turbo-boost" of power. I feel taller, stronger and straighter. The improvement doesn't plateau, it's the gift of a happy body that keeps giving! My shoulders used to be permanently up near my ears, now they are much more relaxed and down where they should be. It's helped my confidence and ability to feel happy and healthy, not just when doing Pilates but every day. I believe everyone can achieve long-term benefits from Pilates.'

HIP TWIST WITH STRETCHED ARMS

Benefits

This exercise opens up the chest, strengthens all the abdominal muscles including the oblique (waist) muscles, and strengthens the quads and hip flexors. The rotation and the stamina it demands will enhance your walking or jogging form. The exercise teaches the torso to stay balanced and still while the legs are circling.

Note: *if you have a back, wrist or elbow problem, please modify — instructions towards the end of the exercise.*

ADVANCED

Method

- Sit up tall on your 'sit bones' and bend your knees, feet flat on the floor.
- Place your hands on the floor behind you, positioned slightly wider than your hips with your fingers facing forwards (or if you find it more comfortable, with your fingers facing outwards).
- Lean back and take your weight on to your hands.

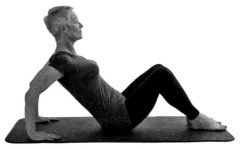

- Engage your abdominal muscles/pelvic floor muscles.
- Raise one leg and lengthen it in front of you, pointing your toes.

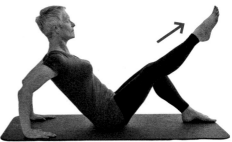

- Raise the other leg to join it, coming into a 'V' position, legs together, toes still pointed.

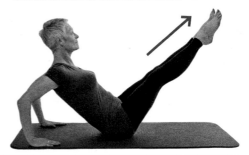

Note:

- Try not to collapse in your centre. Keep lengthened and keep your abdominals engaged throughout, supporting your spine.
- Maintain torso and pelvic stability — don't let them join in and circle with your legs.

- Keep the exercise flowing and try to avoid jerky movements.
- Relax your shoulders; make sure they don't end up around your ears.
- Keep your legs straight, toes pointed and together.
- Breathe!

- Breathe in to prepare.
- Breathe out and slowly begin to circle your legs around to the left side of your body, continuing downwards and then to the other side.

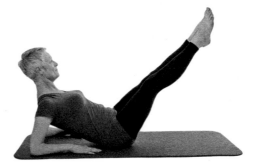

- Start off with a couple of repetitions and then increase, repeating 4 times in one direction and then rotate 4 times the other way. Come into Full Body Stretch.

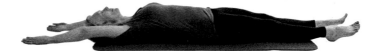

Too challenging for the arms? Try this:
- Perform the exercise while leaning back on your forearms, elbows bent.

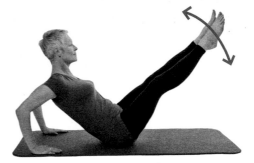

- Take your legs from side to side instead of in a full circle.

- If you attempt the rotations, keep them small until you feel confident that your pelvis isn't moving and your abdominal muscles feel stronger.

CRISS-CROSS

This exercise works the oblique (waist) muscles, as do many of the Side Series exercises (pages 110–118). By strengthening your oblique muscles you will find that there will be less side-to-side twisting when you walk or jog. This twisting often occurs when the body is flagging towards the end of a long walking or jogging session and so wastes precious energy. Take a look at your form the next time you are out and about and see whether you notice any rotational movement. In addition, this exercise is a great core strengthener: it works the lower abdominals, stretches the hip flexors, deep neck flexors, and it improves mobility of the thoracic spine (page 30). It will also improve coordination.

ALL LEVELS

Note: *if you have neck or back problems please take care or modify – instructions towards the end of the exercise.*

Method

- Lie on your back.
- Bend your knees, feet in line with your hips.
- Relax your arms down by your sides.
- Perform a few pelvic tilts to come into Neutral Spine.
- Engage your abdominal muscles/pelvic floor muscles.
- Raise one leg up into Table Top.

- Raise your other leg up into Table Top.
- Place your fingers lightly behind your head, taking your elbows out to the sides, making sure they stay in your peripheral vision.
- Raise your head and your neck off the floor and look towards your knees.

- Breathe in to prepare.
- Breathe out and rotate your ribcage to twist your elbow towards the opposite knee as you extend your other leg out in front of you, pointing your toes.

- Breathe in as you return to centre.
- Breathe out and rotate your torso to the other side, extending the opposite leg away.

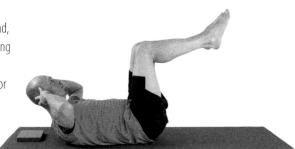

- Repeat up to 10 repetitions, and then if you feel like you could do some more after a rest, repeat the exercise again.
- At the end of the exercise lower your head and neck to the floor and bring your knees into your chest. Give them a hug before returning first one and then the other leg down to the floor. Come into Full Body Stretch.

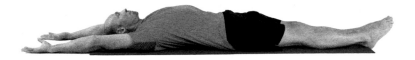

Note:

- Keep your elbows relaxed and wide behind your head – the twist should come from your torso and not just from the elbows. Imagine taking the ribcage across to the opposite hip. Be careful not to drag your head and neck forwards.
- Make sure your shoulders stay up off the floor throughout the exercise.

- Try to keep the movement flowing and use your breathing.
- Maintain pelvic stability and concentrate on keeping your abdominals engaged, extending your legs out in line with your hips.

Too challenging? Try this:

- Perform fewer repetitions.
- Keep your feet on the floor with knees bent throughout the exercise. Curl up towards the knees and then rotate.

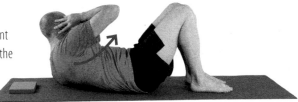

Want more of a challenge? Try this:

- Complete more repetitions.
- Take your legs lower to the ground when you extend, but be very careful that your back doesn't arch if you do so.

THE SAW

Benefits

Like the Dart with Tricep Lift (page 96) and Swan Dive (page 86), this exercise will improve the mobility of the thoracic spine (page 30). This part of the back and shoulders can become tight in our daily activities as the muscles begin to tire and the torso can collapse forwards, especially as we age. These muscles can also be affected by sitting hunched over a desk all day or sitting in a heap on the sofa – I think I might have mentioned this several times before! These muscles, like many others, get tighter as we grow older. The Saw will strengthen and stretch out those back muscles and the rotational movement in this exercise will strengthen the oblique (waist) muscles. You'll also feel a stretch in your hamstrings (back of thighs) and adductor (inside thigh) muscles.

Note: *if you have disc problems, take care with this exercise and make sure rotation is comfortable.*

ALL LEVELS

Method

- Sit up tall on your 'sit bones' and come into Neutral Spine.
- Extend your legs out in front of you, placing them slightly wider than your shoulders. If this is really challenging, see the adaptations that follow on from this exercise.
- Flex your feet for a deeper stretch.
- Take your arms out to the sides of your body, level with your shoulders.

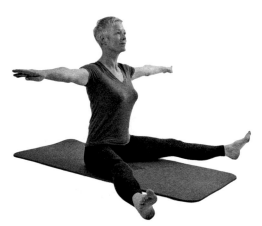

- Engage your abdominal muscles/pelvic floor muscles.
- Breathe in to prepare and slowly rotate your torso to the right.

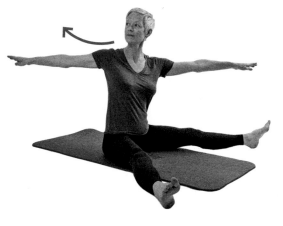

- Breathe out and, taking your chest down towards your leg, reach your left little finger towards your right little toe. Your other arm is lengthened behind your back.
- Breathe in.
- Breathe out as you 'saw' your little finger three times towards and gently against your toe.
- Breathe in.
- Breathe out as you engage your abdominals to lift yourself back up to sitting, lengthening through the spine as you do so.

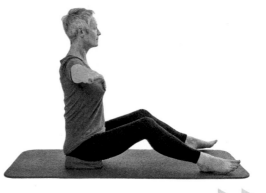

- Breathe in, sitting up tall again.
- Breathe out and repeat to the other side.
- Repeat the exercise 3 times on each side.

Lower back and hamstrings too tight? Try this:
- If sitting with your legs straight out in front of you is not possible, sit on a small cushion or block so that you can sit up tall and not collapse in your centre – this will improve the angle of your pelvis and increase mobility. Alternatively, modify the exercise (see below).

Too challenging? Try this:
- Bend your knees slightly if your hamstrings are really tight, and bring your legs closer together.

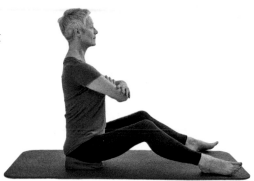

- If your shoulders or arms aren't comfortable being held out to the side, fold them in front of you and just rotate from side to side.
- Decrease repetitions.

Want more of a challenge? Try this:
- Take your legs slightly wider apart but make sure you can still sit up on your 'sit bones' with your legs staying aligned.
- Increase repetitions.

Note:
- Keep your abdominal muscles activated throughout.
- Keep your knees and toes aligned, facing the ceiling, don't let your knees roll in.

- Lift out of your hips as you rotate but make sure you don't rise up off the opposite buttock. The feet shouldn't move and should remain level with each other.

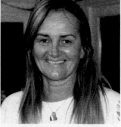

CASE STUDY

Kimberly Patel
Age: 51
Occupation: Office and Heath and Safety manager
Practised Pilates for: 6 years
Favourite exercises: Leg Pull/Plank and Roll Back (pages 88 and 162)

'I've found Pilates has benefited my overall fitness levels. By doing Pilates I have found it has given me more strength in my weak knee and lower back. I am more aware of sitting for long periods of time and I make sure I sit at the correct angle at my work PC and take regular breaks. If I don't attend class, I notice it – so it must be doing me good!'

SPINE TWIST

Benefits

This is a classic mat Pilates exercise that strengthens the oblique (waist) muscles, abdominal and back muscles. It improves spinal mobility, including the head and neck, but especially the thoracic spine. It's a great exercise to help improve circulation and for relieving tension, but requires good abdominal control to keep the spine lengthened and stable as you twist so that you remain sitting upright without slouching. This exercise is more challenging than it looks, so pay particular attention to your spinal alignment.

> Have you warmed up? Return to Chapter 7 for the gentle warm-up exercises.

> **Note:** *if you have disc problems or a back injury, proceed with caution or omit this exercise.*

ALL LEVELS

Method

- Sit up tall on your 'sit bones' and come into Neutral Spine.
- Extend your legs out in front of you along the floor with your feet flexed, placed hip-width apart.
- Take your arms out to the sides with your palms facing downwards.

- Engage your abdominal muscles/pelvic floor muscles.
- Breathe in to prepare as you lengthen through your spine.
- Breathe out as you gently turn to the right and rotate your torso, starting with your head and neck and then through the rest of your spine until you are looking over your shoulder.

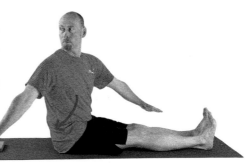

- Hold the position as you breathe in.
- Breathe out and return with control to centre.
- Repeat 5 times each side.

Note:

- Make sure that you are rotating from your waist; engage those abdominals as you move so that your arms just move freely with you – don't use your arms to lead.

- Be aware of any movement in the pelvis and stabilize to avoid it.
- Try not to lean forwards as you twist – your legs should remain still.

Too challenging? Try this:

- Sitting upright on your 'sit bones' and staying in
  Neutral Spine can sometimes be difficult, so sit on a
  small cushion or block to bring yourself into
  the correct position. Or modify the
  position that you sit in for the
  exercise (see below).

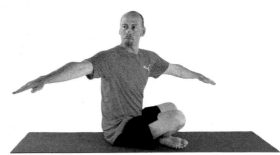

- If sitting with your legs out in front of you and remaining lengthened through the spine while
  maintaining a neutral position is challenging, or your hamstrings are so tight that you can't straighten
  your legs, choose one of the following leg positions:

- legs crossed

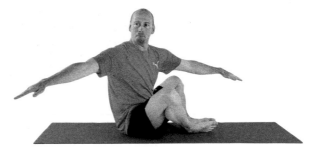

- soles of the feet together

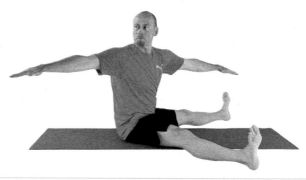

- legs open and fully extended.

- For shoulder problems that make holding your arms out to your sides uncomfortable, place your hands on your shoulders as you twist.

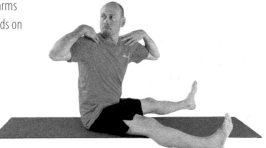

- Or bring your hands together in front of you into a praying position, elbows to the side.

- Alternatively, take your arms to the sides, fingertips/hands to the floor.

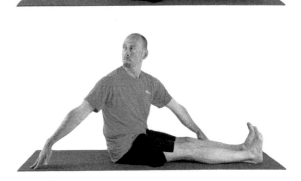

Want more of a challenge? Try this:
- Increase repetitions.
- Increase range of movement and twist further round.

SPINAL MOBILITY AND OBLIQUE STRETCH

Benefits

Although primarily a stretch, this exercise will strengthen the oblique (waist) muscles and so reduce any unwanted twisting in your torso as you walk or jog, which, as mentioned before, can waste precious energy. This exercise is wonderful for the lower back and can be performed as part of your exercise routine or as a post-walk/activity stretch to relieve any lower back tension.

ALL LEVELS

Method

- Lie on your back with your knees bent, feet in line with your hips and your arms stretched out by your sides.

- Perform a few pelvic tilts to come into Neutral Spine.
- Engage your abdominal muscles/pelvic floor muscles.
- Lift your right foot off the floor and inwardly rotate to place your right ankle across your left thigh.

- Breathe in to prepare.
- Breathe out and let your right knee gently drop down to the floor, lifting your left hip as you do so and rotating in the spine.
- Breathe in as you hold the stretch.

- Breathe out, engaging your abdominal muscles as you lift the knee back up to the start position.
- Repeat up to 4 times in total and then change sides.

Too challenging? Try this:
- Take your knee just halfway if you find the stretch too intense.
- Your opposite hip will lift off the floor, but keep the opposite shoulder down on the floor, don't let it join in.

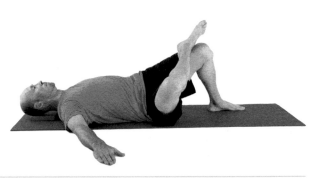

KNEE DROP

Benefits

This is a progression from the knee drop exercise in the Starter Pack (page 74) and so encourages hip mobility and pelvic stability even more, once again challenging the core muscles.

Have you warmed up? Return to Chapter 7 for the gentle warm-up exercises.

Method

- Lie on your back.
- Place a block or small cushion under your head to keep your neck and spine aligned.
- Take your arms out to your sides and keep them relaxed.
- Bend your knees.
- Place your feet in line with your hips.
- Bring your legs together so they are touching.

- Perform a few gentle pelvic tilts and come into Neutral Spine.
- Engage your abdominal muscles/pelvic floor muscles.
- Breathe in to prepare.
- Take your arms to the sides, placed just below your shoulders.
- Breathe in to prepare.
- Breathe out and slowly lower both your knees to one side, with control, to the floor.

- Now extend and lengthen the top leg along the still bent bottom leg.

- Hold the position for a couple of breaths.
- Breathe in and slowly bend the knee back.

- Breathe out and, making sure your abdominal muscles are still engaged, lift both knees back to centre.
- Repeat twice on both sides as long as you're comfortable to do so.

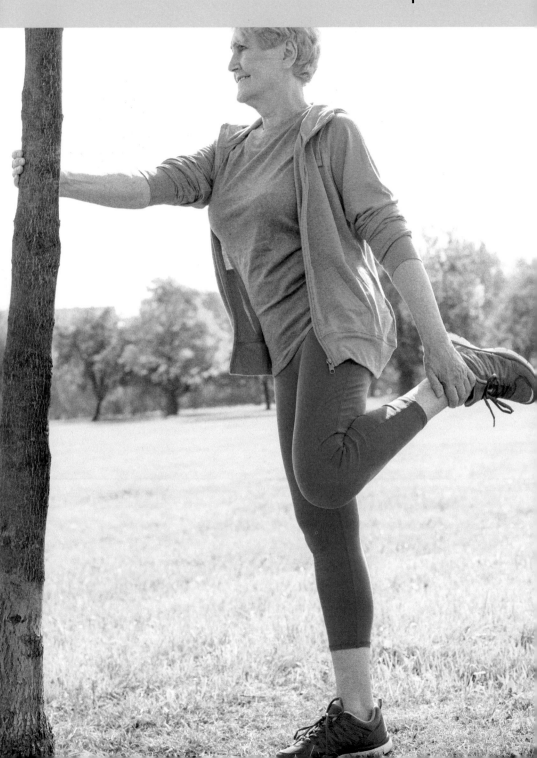

Chapter 11

Post-activity stretches

The following stretches can be performed after the body has warmed up after a long walk, a gardening session, a game of golf or at the end of your Pilates class, or just because your body feels like it could do with a good stretch. This section features a mixture of stretching techniques, some using a Dyna-Band™ and performed on a mat at home, and some standing. The standing stretches are more suitable for when you've come to the end of a long power walk or have been jogging – or even during the walking or jogging session if you feel any muscle tightness.

- Aim to hold the stretch for approximately 20–30 seconds.
- Work within your ability; don't ever force a stretch.
- Only stretch to a point of mild tension, not to pain.
- Stretch slowly.

Note: do not stretch in the first 24–72 hours following an injury, especially if caused by a fall or some kind of trauma. Seek specialist advice if in doubt. Do not bounce in the stretch.

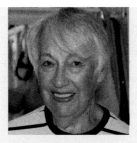

CASE STUDY

Annie Boville
Age: 84
Practised Pilates for: Forever!
Favourite exercise: any stretching exercise and exercises with weights.

'I started Pilates years ago. I do a lot of gardening which I love and want to keep on doing. Pilates particularly helped me after I got new hips and it helped me with back problems. My posture has improved; I stand better, and don't stoop. My core strength, which got less with age, is much improved. It's so important to keep independent in later life and enjoy good health. Pilates definitely contributes to this.'

HAMSTRING, ADDUCTOR AND ABDUCTOR STRETCH WITH DYNA-BAND™

Method

- Lie on your back with knees bent.
- Hold one end of the Dyna-Band™ in each hand.
- Extend your right leg up above your body and hook the centre of your Dyna-Band™ around the sole of your foot.

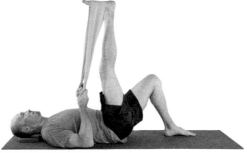

- Engage your abdominal muscles/pelvic floor muscles.
- Breathe in to prepare.
- Breathe out as you gently ease your leg towards your head, feeling a gentle lengthening of the muscles in the back of your thigh.

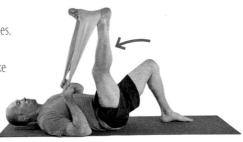

- Breathe naturally and hold for 20–30 seconds.
- Release the stretch and then repeat a couple more times.
- Breathe in.
- Breathe out as you drop your leg to the side – only take it to a comfortable position until you feel the gentle stretch on the inside of your thigh.

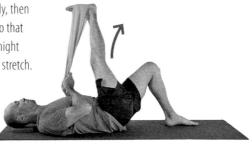

- Breathe naturally and hold the stretch for 20–30 seconds.
- Breathe in.
- Breathe out and lift your leg back up above your body, then let it drop down across the other side of your torso so that you feel a stretch on the outside of your thigh. You might find that you don't have to take it very far to feel the stretch.

- Hold the stretch, breathing naturally for 20–30 seconds.
- Breathe in.
- Breathe out and raise your leg back up to centre.
- Change legs and repeat the whole stretching sequence from the beginning.

GLUTE STRETCH

Method

- Lie on your back with knees bent.
- Place your right ankle across your left thigh.
- Take your right hand between both legs and place it round the inside of your left thigh.
- Place your left hand around the outside of your left thigh.

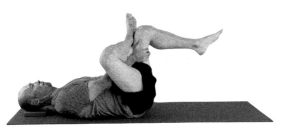

- Engage your abdominal muscles/pelvic floor muscles.
- Raise your head and neck off the floor and look towards your knees.
- Breathe in to prepare.
- Breathe out and slowly pull your left leg towards your chest as you feel a stretch in the buttock area.

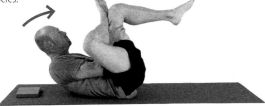

- Breathe naturally and hold the stretch for 20–30 seconds, then release.
- Repeat on the other side.

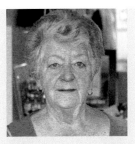

CASE STUDY

Daphne Grube
Age: 74
Practised Pilates for: 12 years
Favourite exercise: Shoulder Bridge (page 146) and arm exercises with weights

'Pilates is definitely keeping me fit and supple which is my prime reason for doing it. I tend to use it as a preventative method to ensure I don't stiffen up as I get older. I'm certainly fit and flexible enough to complete 18 holes of golf two or three times a week.'

STANDING STRETCHES

CALF AND ACHILLES STRETCH

Method

- Stand tall and take your left leg behind you, pressing your heel into the ground.
- Bend your front knee, leaning forwards slightly but keeping your back straight.
- Hold for 20–30 seconds as you feel a lengthening in the back of your calf muscle.

- Change legs and repeat.

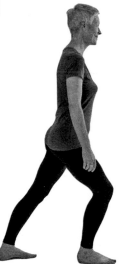

QUADRICEPS AND HIP FLEXOR STRETCH

Method

- Stand tall, engage your abdominal muscles and raise your right foot behind you towards your right buttock.
- Take hold of your foot with your right hand.
- Gently ease your foot and leg with your hand towards your buttock until you feel a gentle stretch in the front of your thigh.

- If you find it hard to balance, hold on to something.
- Try not to arch your back.
- Hold both knees together and tilt your pelvis back for a stronger stretch.

- Hold for 20–30 seconds, breathing naturally, and then change legs.

HAMSTRING STRETCH

Method

- Extend your right leg in front of your left — make sure both knees are parallel.
- Keep your right leg straight and bend your left knee.
- Place your hands on your left thigh for support and make sure you can feel the stretch at the back of your thigh.

- Hold for 20–30 seconds.
- Repeat on the other leg.

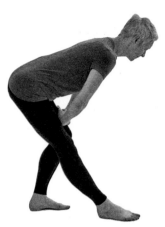

UPPER BACK AND CHEST STRETCH

Method

- Stand tall.
- Raise your arms in front of your chest and 'hug a tree'!
- Hold for about 20 seconds.
- Take your arms behind your back.
- Interlock your fingers and gently raise your arms upwards.

- Hold for 20 seconds.

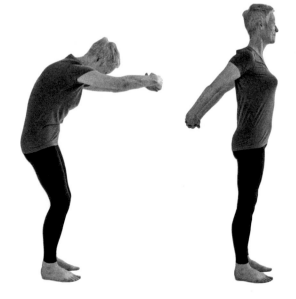

In addition, you could add the following Pilates exercises into your post-walk, gardening, exercise stretching routine:

- Roll Down (page 51)

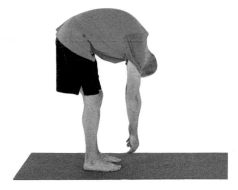

- Cat Stretch (page 77)

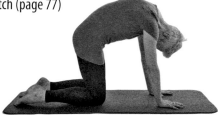

- Chest Opener (page 124)

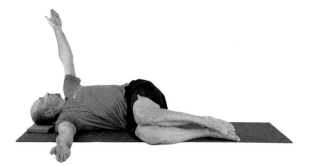

- Extended Child's Pose (page 78)

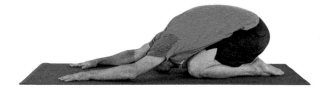

- Cobra Stretch (page 80)

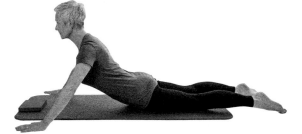

- Hip Roll (page 72)

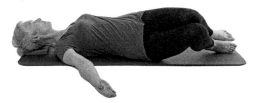

- Spinal Mobility and Oblique Stretch (page 178)

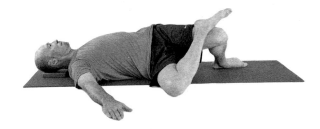

- Shoulder Bridge (page 146)

Chapter 12

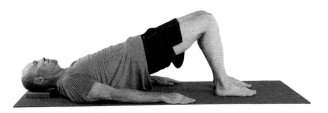

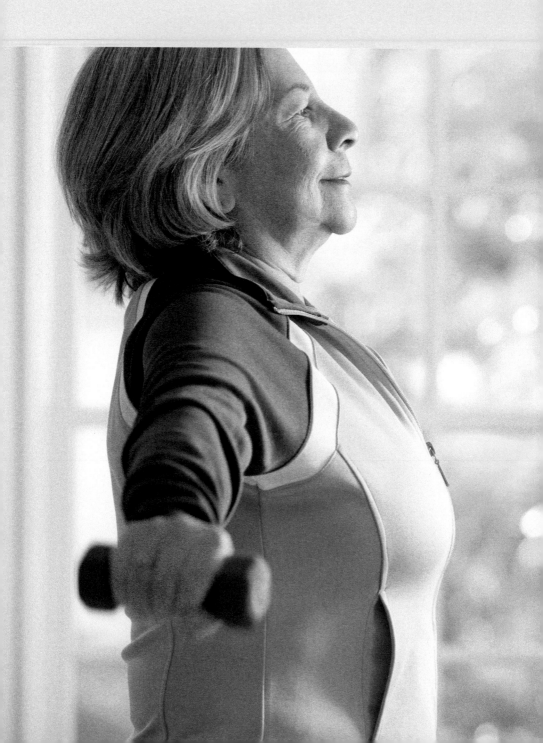

Three 20-minute routines – all levels

Practising some mat Pilates for just 20 minutes every other day, or 10 minutes every day, will pay dividends in the long run. The following are suggested routines to get you into the habit of a regular Pilates practice. To begin with, as you familiarize yourself with the book and the instructions, the routines may, of course, take you longer than 20 minutes. There are too many exercises in the book to include them all here, so just use this as a rough guide to start you off and then add in or remove exercises as you feel necessary. Remember to always perform the Warm-Up (page 44) beforehand, maybe some Balance exercises (Chapter 8) and Foot Strengthening Exercises (Chapter 9), then pick the level that best suits your ability.

Once you're familiar with the exercises you will be able to make up your own exercise sessions. Some days you might want to include more advanced exercises and on others easier ones or just stretches. Experiment, but more than anything, enjoy the process and reap the amazing benefits!

> Make up your mind that you will perform your Pilates exercises for 10 minutes without fail.
>
> Joseph Pilates

BEGINNER

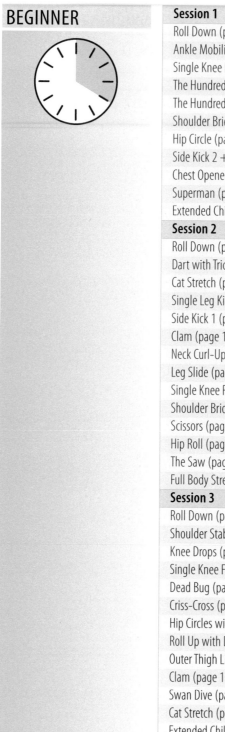

Session 1
Roll Down (page 51)
Ankle Mobility (page 63) + Foot Massage (page 64)
Single Knee Fold (page 126)
The Hundred (preparation) (page 138)
The Hundred (just legs) (page 141)
Shoulder Bridge (page 146)
Hip Circle (page 152)
Side Kick 2 + Inner Thigh (page 112)
Chest Opener (page 124)
Superman (page 92)
Extended Child's Pose (page 78)

Session 2
Roll Down (page 51)
Dart with Tricep Lift (page 96)
Cat Stretch (page 77)
Single Leg Kick (page 100)
Side Kick 1 (page 110) or Single Leg Side Kick (page 75)
Clam (page 119)
Neck Curl-Up (page 70)
Leg Slide (page 68)
Single Knee Fold (page 126)
Shoulder Bridge (page 146)
Scissors (page 158)
Hip Roll (page 72)
The Saw (page 172)
Full Body Stretch (page 81)

Session 3
Roll Down (page 51)
Shoulder Stability (page 130) + Arm Circles (page 134)
Knee Drops (page 179)
Single Knee Fold (page 126)
Dead Bug (page 136)
Criss-Cross (page 170)
Hip Circles with Dyna-Band™ (page 153)
Roll Up with Dyna-Band™ (page 166)
Outer Thigh Lifts (page 120) and Inner Thigh Lifts (page 122)
Clam (page 119)
Swan Dive (page 86) or Swan Dive on Forearms (page 76)
Cat Stretch (page 77)
Extended Child's Pose (page 78)

INTERMEDIATE

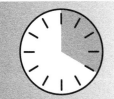

Session 1

Roll Down (intermediate) (page 53)
Swimming into Back Extension (page 85)
Leg Pull/Plank (intermediate) (page 89)
Extended Child's Pose (page 78)
Side Kick 3 into Torpedo (page 114)
Clam (page 119)
Single Knee Fold (page 126)
Neck Curl-Up (page 70)
Single Leg Stretch (page 142)
Shoulder Bridge (page 146)
Hip Roll (page 72)
Full Body Stretch (page 81)

Session 2

Roll Down (page 51)
Shoulder Stability (page 130) + Arm Circles (page 134)
Double Knee Fold (page 128)
Full Body Stretch (page 81)
Dead Bug (page 136)
Scissors (page 158)
Shoulder Bridge (intermediate) (page 147)
Hip Roll (page 72)
Side Kick 2 + Inner Thigh (page 112)
Clam (page 119)
Rotational Cat (page 98)
Leg Pull/Plank (page 88)
Extended Child's Pose (page 78)

Session 3

Roll Down (page 51)
Push Up from Standing (page 104)
Swan Dive (page 86)
Cat Stretch (page 77)
Side Kick 4 + Foreword and Back (page 115)
Chest Opener (page 124)
The Hundred (preparation) (page 138)
The Hundred (page 141)
Hip Circle (page 152)
Roll Up with Spinal Stretch (page 164)
Spine Twist (page 175)
Full Body Stretch (page 81)

ADVANCED

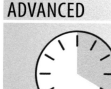

Session 1
Roll Down (intermediate/advanced) (page 53)
Swimming (page 82)
Leg Pull/Plank (advanced) (page 90)
Side Kick 3 into Torpedo (page 114)
Clam (advanced) (page 119)
Single Knee Fold (page 126)
The Hundred (preparation) (page 138)
The Hundred (page 141)
Shoulder Bridge (page 146)
Reverse Leg Pull/Plank (page 155)
Hip Roll (page 72)
Full Body Stretch (page 81)

Session 2
Push Up from Standing (page 104)
Ankle Mobility (page 63)
Double Knee Fold (page 128)
Dead Bug (advanced) (page 137)
Criss-Cross (page 170)
Rolling Like a Ball (page 160)
Hip Twist with Stretched Arms (page 168)
Side Kick 4 + Foreword and Back (page 115)
Clam (advanced) (page 119)
Swan Dive (page 86)
Leg Pull/Plank (page 88)
Extended Child's Pose (page 78)

Session 3
Roll Down (page 51)
Shoulder Stability (page 130) + Arm Circles (advanced) (page 135)
Single Knee Fold (page 126)
The Hundred (preparation) (page 138)
Double Leg Stretch (page 144)
Hip Roll (page 72)
Single Leg Bridge (page 150)
Roll Up with Spinal Stretch (page 164)
Spine Twist (page 175)
Full Body Stretch (page 81)
Side Bend (page 117)
Clam (advanced) (page 119)
Superman (page 92)
Leg Pull/Plank (page 88)
Cat Stretch (page 77)
Extended Child's Pose (page 78)

Chapter 13

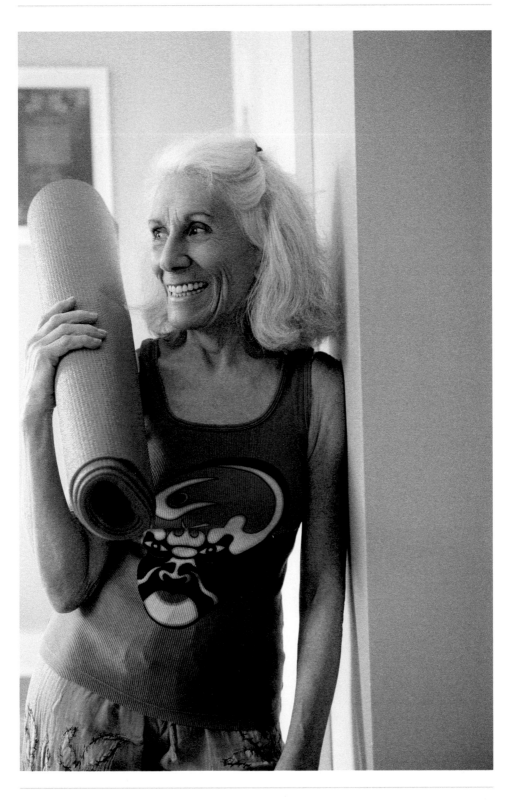

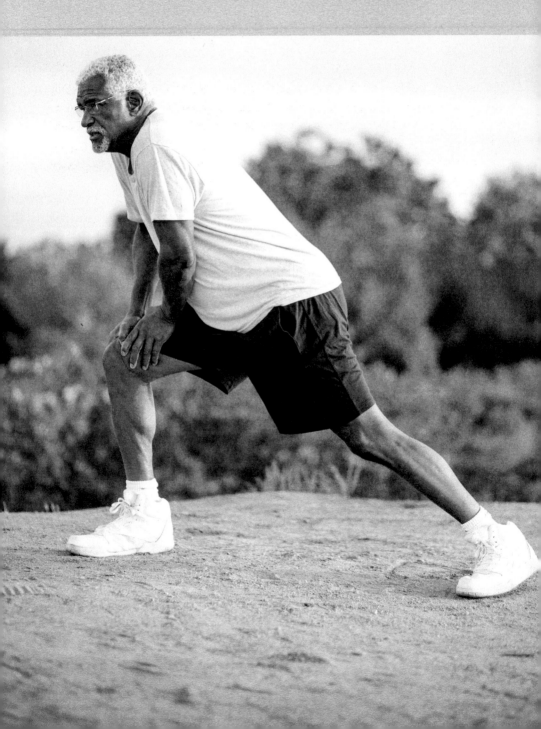

The healing power of Pilates for body and mind

Physical activity can be a life-enhancing experience whatever it is you choose to do and there is no rule that says we have to stop horse riding, playing tennis, golf, or give up jogging or cycling and sit in a chair once we reach a certain age. So, whether or not you're a beginner in your chosen activity or have been involved with some kind of sport all of your life, it is important that we keep fit and healthy enough to continue doing what we love. Sometimes life gets in the way; an illness or a set-back can interrupt the momentum and frailty can be a consequence so we have to reluctantly step back and take time out.

Gentle Pilates exercises can provide calm and healing down-time while you let your body recover. The Starter Pack (page 68) might be all you need to help you begin your journey back to health. The exercises allow you to take stock, rest and give your body and mind the time and resources to recover, so that you can progress on to the other exercises and get back out there to walk those walks, win that tennis match or round of golf, or just be!

The wonderful thing about Pilates is that it puts you in much closer touch with how your body is feeling and functioning. You'll begin to be more aware of minor changes, both mental and physical, during your activities, in a way that you weren't before. As you learn to concentrate and perform the movements in the exercises and get to know your body better, you'll be surprised at how beneficial this form of body conditioning can be on every level.

> A body free from nervous tension and fatigue is the ideal shelter provided by nature for housing a well-balanced mind, fully capable of successfully meeting all the complex problems of modern living.
>
> Joseph Pilates

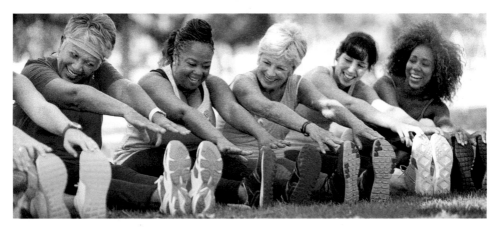

Anyone who exercises, at whatever age, for health, fitness or for fun, knows that a huge part of the challenge can occasionally be just starting your exercise routine of the day or simply getting out of the front door for some fresh air. If the weather is wet and miserable and your 'to do' list feels endless, your joints are feeling a bit achy and you're tired, the challenge is no longer simply a physical one but also mental. Even though the legs might be willing, the sudden lack of motivation can dramatically change your plans and play havoc with fitness levels. Not only that, but once you actually manage to leave the house and start your walk or your round of golf, your mind can sometimes sabotage the enjoyment.

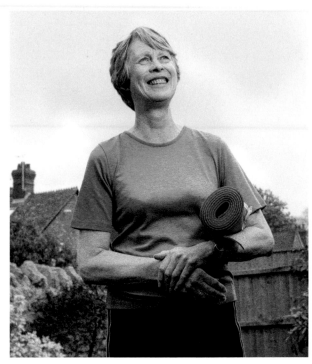

Concentration

This is one of the Pilates principles you have been applying when practising the exercises. When you're playing sport or out and about on a walk, you should be able to focus fully on what you're doing, not allowing any negative thoughts to take over and distract. This can make the difference between playing that winning stroke or feeling completely demotivated and wanting to chuck your golf club into the next sandy bunker.

Even if you're enjoying what started out as a gentle stress-busting, endorphin-filled Sunday morning power walk or game of golf, your mind can suddenly switch to work or family angst and ruin the experience. Keep your conscious mind on the activity, let your unconscious mind sort out all the other stuff. The ability to focus on the right things at the right time is a skill, and by mastering this skill you'll discover that you can play a calmer and more fulfilling game of golf or have a more mindful walk. The knock-on effect is that your body will be happier too. As you learn to concentrate fully on the movements while practising Pilates, together with the balancing and breathing, you will find that your general concentration will improve. The more positive head space that Pilates encourages will also extend into your everyday life which in turn will drive us on as we age.

Meditative walking or even running can be a very life-enhancing and positive thing to practise. Concentrate on your breathing, just as you do when practising the Pilates exercises in this book. Listen to your breathing when you're walking or jogging. Feel it; even count your breaths as a way of centring yourself and distracting your mind from any negative thoughts.

Relaxation

Relaxation is fundamental to our mental and physical health as we age. Research has demonstrated that if you are tense or overly stressed then you are more likely to suffer an injury, to trip when you're out walking or twist an ankle. And of course, the older we are the more prone we are to injury. You might think that you are relaxed, but if your mind is distracted by anxiety then you are likely to be tensing your body. Try to sense any areas of tension – hone in on areas of your body and notice, if, for instance, your fists are clenched or your shoulders are up around your ears when you're out walking. This is where a check on your postural alignment comes into its own. Make sure that you're lengthening through your spine so that you feel lighter on your feet, your chest is wide and open and your shoulders are down and stabilized. All this will have a positive effect on your mind.

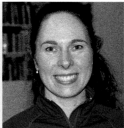

CASE STUDY

Fleur Davey
Age: 46
Occupation: Children and younger person's counsellor
Practised Pilates for: 3 years
Favourite exercises: all of them!

'I have a wonky pelvis – Pilates helps to even me out again after other sports. I notice that if I don't attend a class I have less flexibility in my pelvis and shoulders. I am more aware of my posture, particularly when standing on a moving train, where I like to practise my core strength! Pilates also makes me slow down, physically and mentally – it is my hour of mindfulness.'

Sleep

Like so many other things, our sleep patterns change as we age. Lack of sleep can lead to impaired concentration, memory problems, mood swings and accidents – none of which will help us feel particularly positive about the ageing process. Not to mention how tired it can make us look, which in turn can add on unwanted years. Not good! Sleep is a regenerative process, vital for good health and successful ageing. So what can we do to promote better sleep? Pilates can really help.

There are many well-documented reasons for disturbed sleep. But it's true to say that when we are relaxed and our muscles have been lengthened and gently worked, we have a better chance of sleeping well.

A good night's sleep is something Joseph Pilates wrote about in his book *Return to Life Through Contrology*. He wrote:

'A quiet, cool, well-ventilated room is best. Do not use a soft mattress. "Firm but not soft" is a good rule to follow. Use the lightest possible bed covering consistent with warmth. Do not use large bulky pillows (or as some do, two stacked pillows) – better still, use none at all.'

Many of my clients have told me that, much to their surprise, they sleep better on the day that they practise Pilates as it has a positive, lasting effect. Certainly my own personal experience confirms this too. The breathing we do slows down our heart rate, the lengthening of the muscles allows them to relax and be calm, and the mental focus provides respite from a busy mind. All these factors leave us feeling happy and tired and contribute to a good sleep.

If you've been for a long walk or have been looking after your grandchildren all day, Pilates exercises and stretches will relax your adrenaline-charged body and bring both your mind and body gently 'down' from the exercise or activity high, enabling a better night's sleep and quicker recovery. By the same token if you've been sitting all day, a short Pilates session and stretch before bed is a perfect way to lengthen those tight muscles and get you ready for a good night's sleep.

So if your sleep is disturbed, rise immediately and perform your exercises. It is far better to be tired from physical exertion than be fatigued by "poisons" generated by nervousness while lying awake. Particularly beneficial in this regard are the spinal "rolling" or "unrolling" massage exercises which relax the nerves and induce sound, restful sleep.

Joseph Pilates

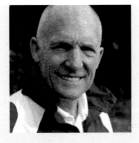

CASE STUDY

Brian Bower
Age: 64
Occupation: Business owner/Manager
Practised Pilates for: 1 year
Favourite exercise: All the stretching exercises

'For me Pilates is the obvious counterbalance to my running – I run a lot of long-distances. Initially, I thought it would just make me stronger and more flexible, which of course it has, but the overriding benefit to me when I attended an evening class was that I relaxed, and consequently my sleep was far deeper and better than it usually was – and my Fitbit proved it!'

Chapter 14

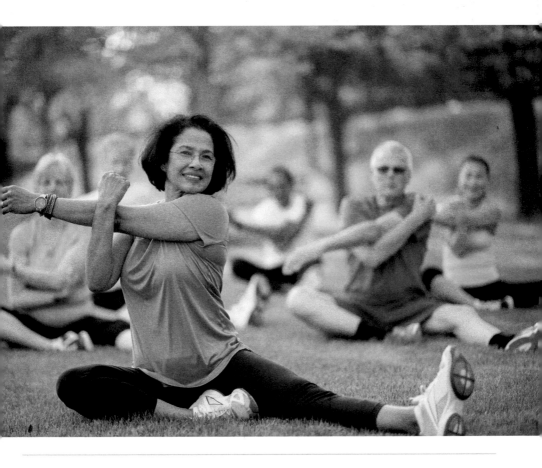

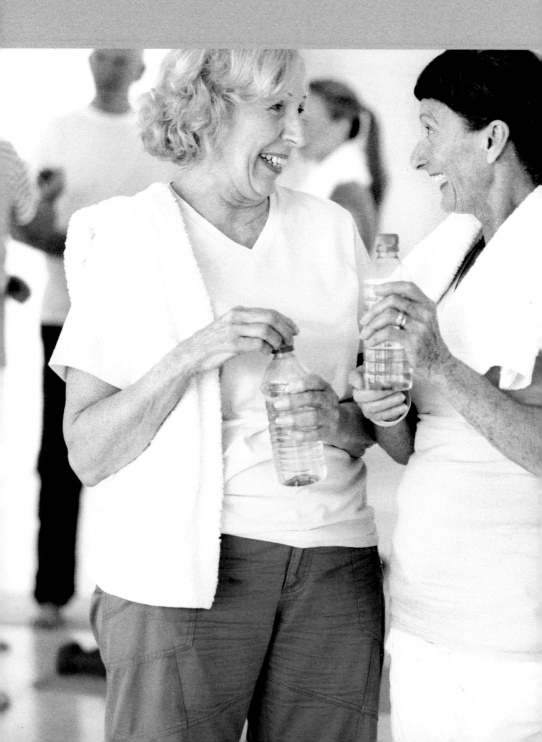

Finding a mat Pilates class and what to look for

All over the world, mat Pilates classes are part of the timetable of every health club, church hall and gym. Sessions are often very popular, but ideally there should be a maximum of about 12 people in each class. The reality these days is that there are a lot more people attending and so often the classes are oversubscribed. Some gyms and health clubs even run Pilates classes designed specifically for the over 50s or 60s.

If you are new to Pilates and have chosen to attend a class, ask the instructor to go through all the posture points with you beforehand to explain the 'Pilates language'. Although I've described everything I think you will need to know, each teacher will have their own way of explaining things. The instructor or health club should automatically check that you have no injuries or musculoskeletal problems and you will be asked to fill in a health questionnaire. If you do have problems, make sure the instructor is familiar with your injury or ailment and is happy to adapt the exercises to suit your individual needs. If your physiotherapist or sports therapist has recommended you try Pilates, it might be helpful for the instructor to have a letter or outline of your problems and what they advise. She/he will also check on what other exercise you do, your fitness level and why specifically you're choosing to come to a Pilates class.

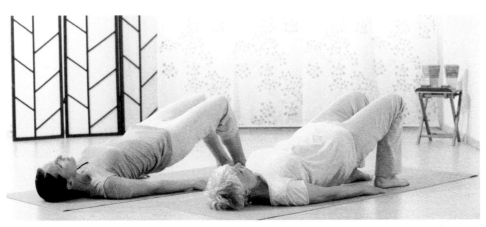

During the class the instructor will stand in different parts of the studio and come round and correct, adjust and attend to you to make sure you are doing the exercises correctly and safely. She/he may demonstrate the exercises but shouldn't be doing them all; his/her cues will be verbal and she/he will be constantly observing.

The first time you attend the class there's often a lot to take in. There may be gentle background music, and there should be space around your mat to move comfortably; you shouldn't feel jammed in like sardines in a tin. Ask questions – never feel you can't. If you don't understand what you're supposed to be doing, say so. A good instructor will welcome this, and often there will be others in the class who might be a tad unsure too and happy that you've spoken up.

Pilates is a wonderful form of exercise and suitable for almost everyone: young, old, athletic, unfit, exercise phobic, but particularly for us as we age. For some, the hardest part is taking the plunge and going along to a class or talking with an instructor for reassurance. Happily, Pilates is at last now attracting more men as they discover the power of this form of exercise. For some men, and I know this from my clients, it's really quite daunting to walk into a class. Joseph Pilates was of course a man and his New York studio was initially mainly frequented by many male boxers, until dancers from the nearby dance studio discovered the amazing powers of his method. He created this extraordinary form of exercise for everyone. So really you have no excuse; equipped with the knowledge and experience gained from this book, all you have to do is sign up for a class. Combine a class and the exercises in this book and you'll be well on your way to living a healthy, happy and active later life.

> I must be right. Never an aspirin. Never injured a day in my life. The whole country, the whole world, should be doing my exercises. They'd be happier.
>
> Joseph Pilates

Glossary

Abductor – your outside thigh muscles.

Achilles tendon – the tendon stretching from the bone of your heel at the back of your leg to your calf muscles that sit just above it.

Adductor – your inside thigh muscles.

Contrology – the original name for Pilates.

Glutes/gluteal muscles – your buttock muscles.

Hamstrings – your back thigh muscles.

Hip flexors – these sit at the top of the thigh/bottom of the torso. They help bring the leg closer to the body.

Iliotibial band (ITB) – the tendon that stretches down the side of your leg from your pelvis to your knee.

Intra-abdominal pressure – pressure within the abdominal cavity when the TVA and pelvic floor muscles work together to support the spine and pelvis during any exertion.

Kinaesthetic sensing – awareness of movement of muscles and joints. Kinaesthetic sense helps control and coordinate activities.

Kyphosis – where the upper back curves excessively and the shoulders are rounded.

Lateral thoracic breathing – breathing into your ribcage.

Lordosis – where there is an excessive curvature or arch of the lower back.

Lumbar spine – the lower back.

Neutral Spine – all Pilates exercises start from Neutral Spine. It is a good, strong healthy position where your spine is lengthened and in its natural curves.

Obliques – your waist muscles.

Open your chest – when your shoulders are back and down, and your chest is wide and open.

Proprioception – the ability to sense the position, location and orientation of your limbs in space.

Quadriceps – your front thigh muscles.

Rectus abdominis – your 'six pack' that sits on top of the TVA.

Scooping the abdominals – when you pull your abdominal muscles in and up.

Sit bones – the bones of the lower pelvis that you sit on.

Soften your shoulder blades/knees/elbows – when you bend them slightly.

Table Top – position of the body when lying on your back, abdominal muscles engaged and either one or both of your legs are raised so that your knee is above your hip and your shin is parallel to the ceiling.

Tensor fasciae latae (TFL) – the muscle located on the outside of the hip above the ITB.

Thoracic spine – the mid-upper back.

Transversus abdominis (TVA) – the deep tummy muscles that wrap around your middle between your lower ribs and the top of your pelvis. These work together with your pelvic floor muscles.

Trapezius – your upper back muscles.

Triceps – the muscles in the back of your upper arm (bingo wings!)

About the Author

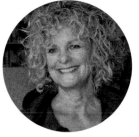

Harri is an experienced REPS Level 3 Pilates instructor. She works out of her private studio in Marlow, Buckinghamshire, where she holds popular weekly mat Pilates classes and sees clients on a one-to-one basis. Pilates should be accessible to all, she believes, and so is passionate about spreading the word and demonstrating how powerful this form of exercise can be for people at all stages of life, particularly as we grow older. She has seen how Pilates can change people's lives for the better – both mentally and physically. In addition to teaching Pilates, she's a personal trainer and a leader in running fitness who loves nothing more than getting out in the fresh air and hitting the trails.

In the 1980s Harri combined a career as an actor with teaching aerobics and body conditioning – at a time when Pilates first appeared in the UK. A time too when Jane Fonda's high impact exercise routines were popular, 'feeling the burn' was a 'buzz-phrase', and pink leg warmers and head bands were compulsory!

Nowadays though, her passion is to motivate the over fifties to get out there, get active and stay active. She leads a running group called Harri's Running Team, known locally as HRT! The thriving group ranges from beginners to marathon runners, of all ages, shapes and sizes – many of whom swear by the power of Pilates!

You can follow her on Twitter or Instagram (@harriangell) or contact her through her websites: www.runwithharri.co.uk or www.harriangell.com.

Acknowledgements

I couldn't have written this book without the wonderful contributions from my Pilates clients – so thank you! Thank you to the experts: Jane Kaushal and Dr Helen Kennedy for their invaluable input. And of course Charlotte, Sarah and the team at Bloomsbury for their support and guidance.

Index

abdominal muscles 16, 30, 34–5, 37
  cat stretch 77
  cobra 80
  criss-cross 170–1
  double leg stretch 144–5
  hip rolls 72
  hip twist with stretched arms 168–9
  the hundred 138–41
  neck curl-up 70–1
  roll backs 162–3
  roll up with spinal stretch 164–5
  rolling like a ball 160–1
  single knee fold 126–7
  single leg stretch 142–3
  spine twist 175–7
  swan dive 86
  swan dive on forearms 76
abductors 115, 120–1, 152
Achilles and calf muscle strengthener 60
Achilles tendon 60, 108
adductor muscles 122, 152, 172
ageing process 7, 8, 9, 15, 35
ankle mobility 63, 115
ankle weights 26
anxiety 29, 31
arm circles 134–5
arm muscles
  arms and shoulders 131
  arms, shoulders and spinal mobility
    132
  dart with tricep lift 96–7
  dead bug 136–7
  leg pull/plank 88–91
  push-up from standing 104–7
  reverse leg pull/plank 155–7
  shoulder stability 130
  single leg kick 100
  swimming (Pilates exercise) 82–4
arthritis 42, 84

back muscles 17
  chest opener 124–5
  dead bug 136–7
  double leg kick 102–3
  the hundred 138–41

reverse leg pull/plank 155–7
roll downs 51
rotational cat 98–9
the saw 172–4
scissors 158–9
shoulder bridge 146–9
shoulder stability 130
single knee fold 126–7
single leg kick 100–1
spinal mobility and oblique stretch
  178
spinal rotations (twisting) 47
spine twist 175–7
swan dive 86
swan dive on forearms 76
swimming (Pilates exercise) 82
back problems 16–17, 30, 41
balance 17, 18, 23, 43, 49, 55–7, 59, 79,
  98–9, 160–1
bone mass 23
brain gym for feet 61
breast surgery 43
breathing 18–19, 22, 39

calf and Achilles stretch 184
calf muscles 60, 72, 88, 108
case studies 18, 29, 53, 65, 69, 71, 81,
  84, 87, 91, 95, 101, 111, 116, 121,
  123, 125, 127, 129, 133, 135, 137,
  140, 151, 161, 163, 167, 174, 181,
  183, 197, 199
cat stretch 77, 186
  into down dog 108–9
  centring 22
chest opening 18, 76, 80, 86, 98, 102,
  124–5, 155, 168, 186
circulation 138
clam (lateral hip opener) 119
clothing 25
cobra stretch 80, 187
concentration 21, 22, 55, 196–7
Contrology 11–12
coordination 17–18, 55, 68–9, 92–5,
  108–9, 142–5, 158–9, 160–1
core muscles 16–17

see abdominal muscles; back muscles;
  glutes/buttocks; hips/hip mobility;
  obliques (waist)
core strength/stability 16, 22, 41
criss-cross 170–1
curl-ups 70

dart with tricep lift 96–7
dead bug 136–7
deltoids 155
diaphragm 18–19, 22, 39
double knee fold 128–9
double leg kick 102–3
double leg stretch 144–5
down dog, cat stretch into 108–9
Dyna-Bands™ 25
  exercises 153, 166, 182

energy levels 18, 19
engaging your muscles 34–5
equipment, Pilates 25–6
erector spinae 17, 92
extended child's pose 78–9, 186

fall prevention 23, 55–7
flexibility 19, 23, 31, 43, 59, 77, 79,
  98–9, 142–5, 164–5
  see also stretching/stretches
flow 23
foam blocks 25
foot health/strengthening 59–64
  Achilles and calf muscle strengthener
    60
  ankle mobility 63
  brain gym for feet 61
  foot massage 64
  heels and toes 62
foot massage 64
foot roller/foot massage ball 25, 64
full body stretch 81

glute stretch 183
glutes/buttocks 16–17
  clam (lateral hip opener) 119
  double leg kick 102–3

double leg stretch 144–5
outer thigh lift 120–1
reverse leg pull/plank 155–7
roll down 51
rolling like a ball 160–1
shoulder bridge 146–9
single leg bridge 150–1
single leg kick 100–1
single leg stretch 142–3

hamstring, adductor and abductor stretch
    with Dyna-Band™ 182
hamstring stretch 185
hamstrings 17
    cat stretch into down dog 108–9
    clam/lateral hip opener 119
    double leg stretch 144–5
    hip circles 152–3
    hip roll 72
    push-up from standing 104–7
    roll down 51
    roll up with spinal stretch 164–5
    the saw 172–4
    scissors 158–9
    shoulder bridge 146–9
    single leg kick 100–1
    single leg stretch 142–3
    swimming (Pilates exercise) 82–4
hand weights 26
heart rate 23
heels and toes 62
high blood pressure 23
hip circles 152–3
hip flexors 29
    see also hips/hip mobility
hip openers 50
hip replacements 41–2
hip rolls 72, 187
hip twist with stretched arms 168–9
hips/hip mobility 49–50
    criss-cross 170–1
    double leg kick 102–3
    double leg stretch 144–5
    hip circles 152–4
    hip drop 179
    hip drop starter 74
    hip rolls 72
    hip twist with stretched arms 168–9
    the hundred 138–41
    leg pull/plank 88–91
    leg slide 68

reverse leg pull/plank 155–7
roll backs 162–3
scissors 158–9
shoulder bridge 146–9
side bends/side plank 117–18
side kick 4 + forward and back
    115–16
side kicks 110–16
single knee fold 126–7
single leg bridge 150–1
single leg kick 100–1
single leg side kick 75
single leg stretch 142–3
swimming (Pilates exercise) 82
the hundred 141
    preparation 138–40

iliotibial band (ITB) 110, 115, 119, 120
imprinted spine 32, 37
incontinence, urinary 35–6
inner thigh exercise 113
    lifts 122–3
    see also adductors
intra-abdominal pressure 16, 35

kinaesthetic sensing 17
knee and hip mobility 49–50
knee drop 179
    starter 74
knee replacement 42
kyphosis 30

lateral flexion/side bends 48
lateral hip opener (clam) 119
lateral thoracic breathing 22, 39
leg muscles see abductors; adductors;
    calf muscles; hamstrings; hips/hip
    mobility; quads
leg pull/plank 88–91
leg slides 68
lordosis 30
lower back problems 16–17, 30
    see also back muscles
lumbar spine 30, 160
lung capacity/health 18, 39, 124

mats, yoga/Pilates 25
menopause 31, 35
mental health/wellbeing 19, 23, 30, 31,
    69, 195–8
mindfulness 21

mirrors 33–4, 44
multifidus 17

neck exercises 45, 70–1, 124–5, 142–3,
    144–5, 170–1
neck flexors 70
neck warm-up 45
neutral spine 22, 32–3, 37

obliques (waist muscles) 16
    criss-cross 170–1
    hip rolls 72
    hip twist with stretched arms 168–9
    the saw 172–4
    send bend 117–18
    side kicks 75, 110–16
    spinal mobility and oblique stretch
        178
    spine twist 175–7
oestrogen deficiency 31, 35
one leg knee fold 73
osteopenia 70
osteoporosis 23, 70, 75
outer thigh lift 120–1

pectoral muscles 104, 124, 155
pelvic floor muscles 16, 22, 34, 35–6
pelvic tilts 32
pelvis/pelvic stability 16, 30, 35, 36
    clam (lateral hip opener) 119
    hip circles 152–3
    the hundred 138–41
    inner left thigh 122–3
    knee drop 179
    knee drop starter 74
    leg pull/plank 88–91
    leg slide 68
    one leg knee fold 73
    reverse leg pull/plank 155–7
    single knee fold 126–7
    single leg bridge 150–1
    single leg side kick 75
    swimming (Pilates exercise) 82–4
Pilates class, finding a 201–2
Pilates, Joseph 7, 8, 11–12, 16, 17, 18,
    19, 34, 35, 189, 195, 198
Pilates principles 21–3
plantar fasciitis 59, 64
post-activity stretches see stretching/
    stretches
post-op exercise 41–2, 43

posture/postural alignment 11, 16, 17,
    18–19, 22, 23, 29–31, 33–4, 41–2
    dart with tricep lift 96–7
    push-up from standing 104–7
    reverse leg pull/plank 155–7
    rotational cat 98–9
    scissors 158–9
    superman 92–5
    swan dive 86–7
power walking 96
precision 22
professional advice 23, 31, 35, 43, 57,
    59, 79
prolapse 35
proprioception 17, 55, 57
push-up from standing 104–7

quadriceps and hip flexor stretch 184
quads 100, 104, 120, 146, 168

rectus abdominals (six pack) 16, 70
relaxation 22–3, 36, 39, 77, 78, 197
reverse leg pull/plank 155–7
roll backs 162–3
roll downs 51–3, 186
roll up with Dyna-Band ™ 166
roll up with spinal stretch 164–5
rolling like a ball 160–1
rotational cat 98
rounded shoulders 29, 30, 86
routines 189
    advanced 192
    beginner 190
    intermediate 191

the saw 172–4
sciatic pain 119
scissors 158–9
shoulder bridges 17, 146–9, 187
shoulders/shoulder stabilization 29,
    36, 46
    arm circles 134–5
    arms and shoulders 131
    chest opener 124–5
    dart with tricep lift 96–7
    extended child's pose 78
    the hundred 138–41
    leg pull/plank 88–91
    reverse leg pull/plank 155–7
    the saw 172–4
    shoulder stability 130

side bend/side plank 117–18
superman 92–5
side bend/side plank 117–18
side kicks
    side kick 2 + inner thigh 112
    side kick 3 into torpedo 114
    side kick 4 + forward and back
        115–16
    side kick 1 110–11
single knee fold 126–7
single leg bridge 150–1
single leg kick 100–1
single leg side kicks 75
single leg stretch 142–3
sleep patterns 23, 198
spinal extensor muscles 92
spinal health 51–2, 56–7, 68–9, 72,
    73, 76, 77, 78, 80, 81, 82–4, 92–5,
    96–7, 98–9, 104–7, 108–9, 132,
    146–9, 155–7, 160–1, 164–65,
    170–1, 172–4, 175–7, 178
    see also back muscles; posture/
        postural alignment; thoracic spine
spinal mobility and oblique stretch 178,
    187
spinal rotation (twisting) 47
spine twist 175–7
stability see balance
stamina 22, 23, 39, 69, 73, 88, 104, 117,
    158, 168
standing tall 33–4
    see also posture/postural alignment
Starter Pack exercises 67
    hip rolls 72
    knee drop starter 74
    leg slides 68–9
    neck curl-ups 70–1
    one leg knee fold 73
    single leg side kicks 75
    swan dive on forearms 76
stress 29
stress relief 23, 31, 84, 95
stretching/stretches 19, 59, 181
    calf and Achilles stretch 184
    cat stretch 77, 186
    chest opener 124, 186
    cobra stretch 80, 187
    extended child's pose 78–9, 186
    full body stretch 81
    glute stretch 183
    hamstring, adductor and abductor

stretch with Dyna-Band™ 182
    hamstring stretch 185
    hip rolls 72, 187
    quadriceps and hip flexor stretch 184
    roll down 51, 186
    shoulder bridges 146–9, 187
    spinal mobility and oblique stretch
        178, 187
    upper back and chest stretch 185
    see also warm-ups
superman 92–5
swan dive 86–7
    on forearms 76
swayback posture 30
swimming (Pilates exercise) 82–4
    into back extension 85

table top position 37, 73
tensor fasciae latae (TFL) 110, 119
thoracic spine 30, 76, 86, 98, 124, 170,
    172
torso strength/stability 15–16, 17,
    22, 35, 68–9, 82–4, 92–5, 114,
    126–7, 134–5, 136–7, 146–9,
    158–9, 168–9, 172–4, 178
transversus abdominals muscle (TVA) 16,
    22, 30, 34–5, 36
trapezius 130
triceps 96, 104

upper back and chest stretch 185

visualization techniques 34–5

waist muscles (obliques) see obliques
    (waist muscles)
walking see posture/postural alignment
warm-ups 33, 44–50, 81
    hip openers 50
    the hundred (preparation) 138–40
    knee and hip-mobility 49
    lateral flexion (side bends) 48
    neck 45
    roll downs 51–3
    shoulders 46
    spinal rotation 47
weight gain 31
weights 26

yoga/Pilates mats 25
yoga straps 25

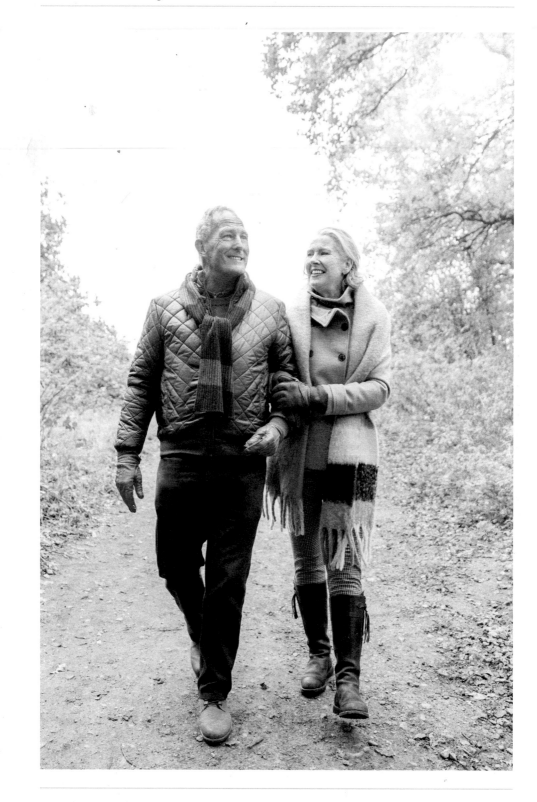